ARTERIOVENOUS FISTULAS-DIAGNOSIS AND MANAGEMENT

Edited by **Stavropoula I. Tjoumakaris**

Arteriovenous Fistulas-Diagnosis and Management

http://dx.doi.org/10.5772/50823
Edited by Stavropoula I. Tjoumakaris

Contributors

Akram Asbeutah, Xianli Lv, Stavropoula I. Tjoumakaris, André Brito Queiroz, Grace Carvajal Mulatti, Erasmo Simão Da Silva, Hede Yan, Weiyang Gao, Feng Zhang, Cunyi Fan, Yasutaka Baba, Iftikhar Ahmad, Shinji Yamamoto, Mohammad Rasouli, Vafa Rahimi-Movaghar, Alexander Vaccaro, Antoine Nachanakian, Fadi Tannouri, Antonios Georges El Helou, Moussa Alaywan, Ghassan Abi Chedid, Bharat Guthikonda

Published by InTech

Janeza Trdine 9, 51000 Rijeka, Croatia

Publishing Process Manager Oliver Kurelic
Typesetting InTech DTP Team
Cover InTech Design Team

Additional hard copies can be obtained from orders@intechopen.com

Arteriovenous Fistulas-Diagnosis and Management, Edited by Stavropoula I. Tjoumakaris
p. cm.
ISBN 978-953-51-1178-8

For EU product safety concerns:
IN TECH d.o.o., Prolaz Marije Krucifikse Kozulić 3, 51000 Rijeka, Croatia, info@intechopen.com or visit our website at intechopen.com.

Meet the editor

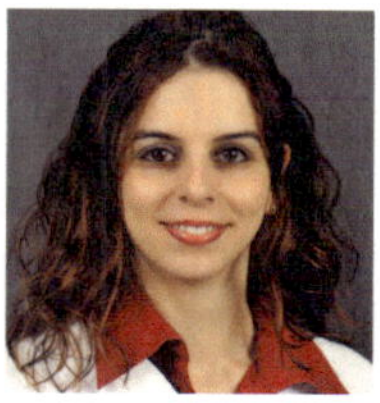

Stavropoula I. Tjoumakaris, MD, is originally from Thessaloniki, Greece. She graduated in Biology with Minors in Physics and Chemistry from Richard Stockton College, Pomona, New Jersey, with Distinction and earned Class Salutatorian Highest Honors. She obtained her medical degree from Jefferson Medical College in Philadelphia, Pennsylvania and received numerous academic distinctions including membership in the prestigious Alpha Omega Honor Society. She completed her Neurological Surgery Residency and advanced Fellowship training in Cerebrovascular Surgery and Endovascular Neurosurgery at Thomas Jefferson University Hospital. She is one of the first and few dual-trained female Cerebrovascular Neurosurgeons in the United States. Dr. Tjoumakaris has been recognized throughout her academic career for both scholastic excellence and a genuine devotion to patient care. She has authored over 100 peer-reviewed articles and book chapters and has lectured internationally on cerebrovascular surgery. She is an Assistant Professor of Neurosurgery at Thomas Jefferson University Hospital and Associate Residency Program Director. Dr. Tjoumakaris is a leader in the diagnosis and management of stroke, aneurysms, arteriovenous malformations and cerebrovascular disease.

To my loving husband, Sidney, and beautiful children Yianni and Scarlett: the joys of my life.
To my mother and best friend, Marika, whose selfless nature and unconditional love truly inspire me.
To my father, Ioannis, a talented physician and even greater father.
To Dr. Robert H. Rosenwasser, my mentor in Neurosurgery and consummate leader.

Contents

Preface

While a relatively uncommon entity, Arteriovenous fistulas represent tremendous challenges to surgeons and patients alike. The condition is as unique as it's multifactorial etiology and multidisciplinary reach.

With this thought in mind, "Arteriovenous Fistulas: Diagnosis and Management", is an attempt to re-visit the basics of this vascular disorder and re-acquaint the reader with the crucial elements of a thorough diagnostic workup and treatment application. Inside this thorough text you will find an inclusive guide to a complete review of the most common presentations of arteriovenous fistulas, the techniques for accurate diagnosis as well as treatment pearls. For simplicity sake, we have divided the text into five major forms of arteriovenous fistulas: 1) Intracranial 2) Spinal 3) Systemic 4) Traumatic and 5) Iatrogenic.

"Arteriovenous Fistulas: Diagnosis and Management" takes complex subject matter and distills it to an easily understood, reproducible and enjoyable experience that will be welcomed by surgeons across subspecialties, including Neurological, Orthopaedic, Vascular, Trauma and General, as well as non-surgeons such as Neurologists and Critical Care Intensivists. Attendings, fellows, residents, medical students or anyone interested in sharpening their diagnostic and therapeutic skill set will benefit from reading this text.

Finally, I must thank all of the authors who contributed so much of their time, wisdom and experience in creating the final product you hold before you. On behalf of everyone associated with this work, I sincerely hope you enjoy learning and implementing your new skills as much as I have enjoyed organizing the material.

Stavropoula I. Tjoumakaris, MD
Assistant Professor
Department of Neurological Surgery
Thomas Jefferson University Hospital
Philadelphia, Pennsylvania

Section 1

Intracranial Arteriovenous Fistula

Chapter 1

Endovascular Management of Dural Arteriovenous Malformations

Nohra Chalouhi, Pascal Jabbour, Aaron S. Dumont, L. Fernando Gonzalez, Robert Rosenwasser and Stavropoula Tjoumakaris

Additional information is available at the end of the chapter

http://dx.doi.org/10.5772/55219

1. Introduction

1.1. Classification systems and prognosis of DAVM

DAVM are typically classified by location of the involved sinus or shunt as well as by the pattern of venous drainage. [5] The pattern of venous drainage is a key factor predicting the natural history of these lesions and provides the foundation for the widely adopted Borden [7] and Cognard [8] classification systems. Borden type I DAVM are mostly benign lesions that exhibit normal antegrade flow into a dural sinus. Type II lesions exhibit a degree of AV shunting exceeding the capacity of antegrade outflow from the involved sinus resulting in retrograde venous drainage into cortical veins. Type III lesions drain exclusively into cortical veins or a trapped sinus segment (sinus thrombosis at both ends from high-flow venous congestion). The Cognard classification is a modified version of the Djindjian classification and identifies five types of DAVM based on the pattern of venous outflow. Briefly, type I lesions exhibit normal antegrade flow into a dural sinus. Type II DAVM show retrograde venous drainage into the adjacent sinus segments (type IIa), cortical veins (type IIb) or both (type IIa +b). Types III and IV DAVM drain directly into cortical veins, either with (type IV) or without (type III) venous ectasia. Type V DAVM are typically localized to the tentorium or dural coverings of the posterior fossa and are further characterized by drainage inferiorly into spinal perimedullary veins.

Both classification systems have been validated and appear to correlate well with the risk of intracranial hemorrhage or non-hemorrhagic neurologic deficit (NHND). [9] Borden types II and III DAVM are associated with a more aggressive natural history and when technically feasible are generally treated because of their increased risk of symptomatic presentation. In a study that included 20 patients with Borden type II and III lesions, Duffau et al [10] found that rebleeding within 2 weeks after the first hemorrhage occurred in as many as 35% of patients and noted that rehemorrhage carried a worse prognosis than the initial hemorrhage. The authors recommended complete and early treatment of ruptured DAVM with cortical venous drainage (CVD). On the other hand, Borden type I DAVM generally have a benign natural history. In a study where 68 patients with Borden Type I DAVM were conservatively treated and followed for a mean of 27.9 months, Satomi and colleagues [11] found that only 1 patient suffered an intracranial hemorrhage and noted a benign and tolerable level of disease in 98.5% of cases. However, according to a recent report, the risk of conversion of a Type I lesion to a more aggressive lesion with CVD appears to be higher than previously reported (annual rate of 1%). [12] Any change in patient symptoms should therefore prompt repeat angiographic imaging to rule out the development of alternative drainage routes.

The annual risk of hemorrhage of DAVM varies between 1.8% and 15%. [13-14] The first hemorrhagic episode of a DAVM is associated with >30% mortality or serious disability.

The annual mortality rate for DAVM with CVD may be as high as 10.4% with a combined annual risk of intracranial hemorrhage and NHND of 15%. [15] Recent data suggest that the natural history of DAVM dependents not only on the pattern of venous drainage, but also on the mode of presentation. As such, Soderman et al [16] found that the annual hemorrhage risk of Borden Type II or III DAVM was 7.4% for patients presenting with intracranial hemorrhage compared with only 1.5% for those with non-hemorrhagic presentation. Likewise, in a study by Strom et al [17] that included 28 patients with Borden Type II or III DAVM, the risks of hemorrhage and NHND were 7.6% and 11.4% respectively for lesions with symptomatic CVD versus only 1.4% and 0% for those with asymptomatic CVD. Based upon these data, Zipfel et al [18] proposed the inclusion of the mode of presentation (symptomatic or asymptomatic CVD) into the Borden and Cognard classification systems to allow for more accurate risk stratification in patients with high-grade DAVM.

Type	Borden	Cognard
I	Drains directly into venous sinus or meningeal vein	Normal antegrade flow into dural sinus
II	Drains into dural sinus or meningeal veins with retrograde drainage into cortical veins	a) Retrograde flow into sinus(es) b) Retrograde filling of cortical vein(s) a+b) Retrograde drainage into sinus(es) and cortical vein(s)
III	Drains into cortical veins without dural sinus or meningeal involvement	Direct drainage into cortical veins without venous ectasia.
IV		Direct drainage into cortical veins with venous ectasia >5 mm and 3x larger than diameter of draining vein.
V		Drainage to spinal perimedullary veins

Table 1. The Borden and Cognard classification systems of DAVM

More recently, Geibprasert et al [19] have proposed an ambitious classification, conceptually unifying pathophysiologic consequences of cranial and spinal DAVM on an embryologic basis. The scheme is based on the venous afferent patterns of three epidural spaces: 1) the ventral drainage group derived from the notochord and corresponding sclerotome extending from the base of the sphenoid to the sacrum, 2) the dorsal epidural space derived primarily from the dorsally located intracranial dural sinuses as this space is not well-developed in the spine, and 3) the lateral epidural shunts located where lateral pial emissary bridging veins pierce the dura. By examining 300 patients with DAVM and categorizing their lesions by their respective afferent venous patterns, Geibprasert et al were able to establish some clinical generalizations about each group. Ventral epidural shunts demonstrated a 2.3:1 female predominance and were less likely associated with cortical venous reflux unless there was extensive thrombosis of the epidural drainage or an especially high-flow shunt. Similarly, dorsal epidural shunts were less likely to reflux into the cortical veins unless thrombosis was present. These lesions did not demonstrate sex predominance but did tend to occur in a lower age group (pediatric) and more frequently occur as multiple lesions. The lateral epidural shunts tended to present in older patients and were more common in men. These lateral lesions were always clinically aggressive and demonstrated significant cortical venous reflux.

2. Clinical features of DAVM and anatomic considerations for embolization

The clinical features associated with DAVM generally depend on the location of the lesion, the extent of the AV shunting, and associated abnormalities of venous drainage. [20-21] Symptoms may be indistinguishable from those associated with pial brain arteriovenous malformations and may include headache, diplopia, blurred vision, or neurologic dysfunction. Focal neurologic deficits and seizures may develop in relation to disturbances in regional cortical venous drainage resulting from the redirection of venous flow from the shunt into pial veins, potentially congesting venous territory remote from the site of the dural fistula. In patients with severe compromise of the deep venous drainage of the brain or with diffuse intracranial hypertension resulting from the obstruction of both sigmoid sinuses, the clinical presentation may include dementia. [5] Dementia may also develop in patients with superior sagittal sinus DAVM due to venous congestion of bilateral frontal lobes. Closure of the arteriovenous shunts may successfully reverse this state only when there are adequate residual venous channels available for the normal venous drainage of the brain. Rarely, cranial neuropathy or unilateral visual phenomena may arise secondary to arterial steal without evidence of associated venous hypertension. [22] Focal symptomatology may worsen or change as a result of the redirection of venous outflow from a DAVM. For example, progressive thrombosis and occlusion of the inferior and superior petrosal sinuses may be associated with worsening of signs in a patient with a cavernous sinus DAVM draining anteriorly through the ipsilateral ophthalmic veins. If contralateral drainage is available, the venous sinus hypertension may be transmitted to the contralateral cavernous sinus, leading to development of bilateral orbital symptoms.

The signs and symptoms of increased intracranial pressure occasionally complicate cases of DAVM. In certain cases this can be attributed to diminished CSF absorption through the arachnoid villi resulting from the transmission of increased venous pressure throughout the superior sagittal sinus. Patients may present with typical symptoms of normal pressure hydrocephalus, such as progressive dementia, gait disturbance, and urinary incontinence. [23] Alternatively, obstruction of the cerebral aqueduct secondary to compression of the mesencephalon by an ectatic draining vein may occur, leading to obstructive hydrocephalus. [24]Moreover, aneurysmal venous ectasia may unusually cause symptomatic mechanical compression of adjacent neurologic structures, most commonly in DAVM draining into pial veins of the posterior fossa. This is particularly true for type IV DAVM, which not infrequently present with clinical symptoms related to mass effect caused by pronounced venous ectasia. [5]

Approximately 20 to 33 percent of patients with symptomatic DAVM present with an intracranial hemorrhage. This most frequently is encountered in lesions involving the floor of the anterior cranial fossa or the tentorium cerebelli; however, it may occur in any case associated with cortical venous drainage, particularly in the presence of significant cerebral venous ectasia.[2] In a recent large study by Bulters et al, [25] DAVM associated with venous ectasia had a 7-fold increase in the incidence of hemorrhage (3.5% no ectasia vs 27% with ectasia). Therefore, patients with venous ectasia may represent a high-risk group that requires rapid intervention.

For those DAVM that present in ways other than hemorrhage, the clinical presentation depends entirely on the grade, location and venous afferent pattern of the fistula. This allows DAVM to be categorized clinicoanatomically into those involving the cavernous sinus, transverse and sigmoid sinuses, superior sagittal sinus, petrosal sinus, torcular, tentorial incisura, and anterior cranial base.

Approximately one-third to one-half of symptomatic intracranial DAVM involve the transverse and sigmoid sinuses. [26] Nearly half present with a subjective bruit as the first clinical manifestation due to proximity of the draining sinus to the middle ear. The tinnitus is synchronized to arterial pulsations and results from increased blood flow into the sigmoid or transverse sinuses. Auscultation over the retroauricular area usually reveals the pulsatile bruit. As with the other DAVM, additional neurologic symptoms and findings generally depend on the pattern of venous drainage encountered in the individual patient. Symptoms may include chronic signs of increased intracranial pressure potentially leading to papilledema and optic atrophy in addition to disturbances related to balance and hearing. Aggressive neurologic symptoms may occur in up to 27% of patients with transverse and sigmoid DAVM. In progressive cases, associated with obstruction of the ipsilateral jugular outflow redirected venous drainage into pial veins of the posterior fossa may result in brain stem or cerebellar dysfunction as well as posterior fossa hemorrhage. Rerouting of drainage into the supratentorial cortical venous compartment may be associated with the development of focal neurologic deficit or seizures as well as increased risk of intracranial hemorrhage. Spontaneous occlusion of transverse and sigmoid DAVM is rare (5%) and generally occurs after hemorrhagic events.

http://dx.doi.org/10.5772/55219

DAVM involving the superior sagittal sinus, tentorial incisura, petrosal sinuses, and anterior cranial base occur less frequently than DAVM involving the transverse, sigmoid, or cavernous sinuses. [5, 27] In these lesions, symptoms typically depend on the route of abnormal venous drainage and associated pattern of venous hypertension, and may include dysphasia, hemiparesis, hemisensory deficits, and abnormal visual phenomena. Several specific features deserve particular attention. (1) Dural fistulas involving the floor of the anterior cranial fossa are usually associated with drainage into ectatic parasagittal cortical veins and often present with intracranial hemorrhage. [27] Moreover, these patients may exhibit unilateral visual loss secondary to arterial steal from the ophthalmic circulation into ethmoidal and recurrent meningeal supplies to the shunt. Although a majority of these lesions are treated with open surgery, embolization through the ophthalmic artery can be undertaken with a reasonably high success rate and low complication risks. [28] (2) DAVM of the petrosal sinuses or tentorial incisura may occasionally drain inferiorly into perimedullary veins of the spinal cord (type V), resulting in progressive myelopathy similar to that encountered in spinal dural AVMs. [26] Assuming the venous sinus drainage of the brain is otherwise unimpaired, these symptoms usually respond well to endovascular or surgical closure of the shunt. Tentorial DAVM drain only via the leptomeningeal-cortical venous system. Consequently, they behave aggressively with severe hemorrhagic and nonhemorrhagic symptoms occurring in 19% and 10% of cases per year. Also, it is not uncommon for such lesions to cause fatal bleeding in the posterior fossa. Therefore, they should be treated aggressively by endovascular and/or surgical means to disconnect the venous drainage system and minimize the risk of hemorrhage and NHND. Superior sagittal sinus DAVM are frequently associated with restrictive change of the superior sagittal sinus and retrograde CVD. Thus, aggressive neurologic symptoms are common and occur in nearly one-half of cases. [29]

DAVM most frequently involve the transverse sinuses. Arterial supply to fistulae of this region predictably derive from identifiable supratentorial and infratentorial sources. The supratentorial group is usually organized around 1) contributors to the basal tentorial arcade, typically including the petrosal and petrosquamosal divisions of the MMA and the lateral division of the meningohypophyseal trunk off the ICA, and, occasionally 2) tranosseous branches of the posterior auricular artery. The infratentorial group commonly involves the jugular division of the ascending pharyngeal artery, transmastoid and more distal transosseous branches of the occipital artery, and the posterior meningeal arteries and artery of the falx cerebelli, either of which can variably arise from the occipital, vertebral or ascending pharyngeal arteries as well as rarely directly from the PICA. With higher flow lesions indirect contribution from contralateral sources may be seen but this usually involves anastomosis with one of the abovementioned conduits as a final common pathway.

In terms of embolization hazards, the petrosal branch of MMA notably gives rise to a branch which anastomoses with the stylomastoid branch of the occipital or posterior auricular arteries forming an arterial arcade within the facial canal which if aggressively embolized (inadvertently) may result in damage to the facial nerve. In that the petrosal branch of the MMA usually participates in the supply of transverse sinus DAVM through the basal tentorial arcade, its contribution to the lesion commonly can be indirectly devascularized by accessing the basal tentorial arcade posterolaterally through the petrosquamosal division of the MMA avoiding the need for direct catheterization and embolization of the petrosal branch altogether. The basal tentorial arcade is an arterial network extending along the insertion of the tentorium into the petrous ridge from the petroclinoid ligament laterally to the transverse sinus. The jugular division of the APA enters the cranial vault via the jugular foramen supplying CN 9,10,11 before dividing into medial and lateral divisions. The medial division courses along the inferior petrosal sinus where it supplies CN 6 and anastomoses with the medial division of the lateral clival branch of MHT. The lateral division runs superiorly along the sigmoid sinus and vascularizes the dura along the transverse sigmoidal confluence. In very high flow fistulae of the distal transverse sinus or lesions of the sigmoid sinus and foramen magnum, recruitment of supply through the hypoglossal division of the ascending pharyngeal artery may be seen (particularly where this artery gives rise to the ipsilateral posterior meningeal artery. Trans-arterial embolizations through this division of the APA (particularly with liquid embolic agents) may result in injury to CN 12 leading to ipsilateral paresis of the tongue.

DAVM of the cavernous sinus (CSDAVM) are most commonly seen in female patients and generally associated with orbital signs and symptoms that fluctuate depending on alterations in orbital venous outflow, which develop secondary to thrombosis and changes in head position. Patients typically present with the gradual onset of focal or diffuse chronic eye redness distinguishable from uveitis. Close inspection reveals dilated tortuous conjunctival and epibulbar vessels that exhibit an acute angulation near the ocular limbus. [30-31] These lesions are often associated with an elevation of episcleral venous pressure leading to a persistent rise in intraocular pressure in the affected eye, potentially resulting in the development of glaucoma. If both cavernous sinuses become involved in the venous drainage secondary to a change in the ipsilateral venous outflow of the affected cavernous sinus, the ocular findings may become bilateral. The patient may complain of pulsatile tinnitus, and in 25 percent of cases a bruit can be auscultated over the orbit. [5] Cranial neuropathies, most commonly involving the sixth nerve, frequently lead to ocular motor dysfunction, which also may be exacerbated by orbital venous congestion and proptosis. More important to the planning of embolization are the hypoxic ischemic retinal changes that develop in approximately 15 percent of patients. [21] Rarely, if thrombosis in the cavernous sinus is extensive, abnormal drainage into cerebral veins may occur, increasing the likelihood of an intracranial hemorrhage or venous infarction. [5] Unfortunately, frequently cited classification schemes of intracranial DAVM are deficient in their handling of CSDAVM due to the lack of explicit consideration given to ophthalmic venous drainage and the clinical consequences of orbital venous congestion. Despite the lack of a coherent classification scheme for CSDAVM, the implications of venous outflow from these lesions are similar to DAVM at other locations and the analysis of venous drainage is important in understanding the pathophysiology of the disease at this site. An excellent study of the clinical manifestations in 85 patients with CSDAVM relative to their angiographic characteristics was reported by Stiebel-Kalish et al. [32-33] In this study, the clinical symptoms found in patients with CSDAVM were related to the abnormal venous drainage and could be predicted by analysis of the aberrant venous drainage patterns. Interestingly, central nervous system symptoms or dysfunction, were found in 7 (8%) of these patients, attesting to the potential danger of cortical venous drainage even among patients with CSDAVM. Spontaneous regression of CSDAVM is a well-described phenomenon that is observed in 10%–50% of cases. [29]

The vascular supply to the dura of the cavernous sinus is complex because of extensive regional anastomoses between dural branches of the internal carotid and branches of the internal maxillary artery (middle meningeal, and accessory meningeal arteries, and the artery of the foramen rotundum). Moreover, the ophthalmic artery may participate indirectly via a tentorial branch of the recurrent meningeal artery. From the perspective of angiographic workup and embolization, these lesions may be divided conceptually into two groups: (1) an anterolateral group, arising from the orbital apex and lateral cavernous sinus, and (2) a posterior group, including the posterior cavernous sinus, petroclinoid ligament, and dorsum sella.

The meningeal supply to anterior division lesions may be considered to reflect the hemodynamic balance between branches arising from the horizontal segment of the cavernous internal carotid artery, most notably the inferolateral trunk (ILT) and meningeal branches of the internal maxillary artery. This latter group includes cavernous and recurrent tentorial branches of the MMA, cavernous meningeal branches of the accessory meningeal artery, and the artery of the foramen rotundum. As expected, embolization of these meningeal arteries should be preceded by superselective angiographic analysis to prevent inadvertent embolization into the internal carotid artery or possible damage to the orbit or regional cranial nerves.

The supply to posterior division lesions is derived primarily from medial and lateral clival (meningohypophyseal) branches of the internal carotid artery and their potential anastomotic connections with branches of the ascending pharyngeal and middle meningeal arteries. These most notably include the ascending clival and inferior petrosal arcades, derived from the hypoglossal and jugular divisions of the ascending pharyngeal artery, respectively; the posterior cavernous branches of the MMA; and the basal tentorial arcade supplied by the petrosal and the petrosquamosal branches of the MMA.

Three critical points should be considered before embolization of fistulae involving this territory. (1) The vascular supply to the intrapetrous facial nerve should be determined. This may arise primarily from the petrous branch of the MMA. For this reason, petroclinoid lesions supplied by the basal tentorial arcade should be embolized preferentially from the petrosquamosal branch of the MMA, thereby avoiding the proximal petrosal artery. (2) Potential contributions from the contralateral internal carotid and ascending pharyngeal arteries via transclival anastomoses should be evaluated, particularly in lesions involving the dorsum sellae. (3) Because embolization of upper clival and petroclinoid lesions may involve the hypoglossal or jugular division of the ascending pharyngeal artery, attention must be directed to the possibility of iatrogenic lower cranial neuropathy when using NBCA, Onyx, or ethanol. Midline lesions requiring aggressive embolization of pedicles from both ascending pharyngeal arteries should be performed as a staged procedure on different days, specifically to avoid development of bilateral hypoglossal nerve deficits.

The simplest and most commonly utilized route to access the cavernous sinus is through the inferior petrosal sinus. Guidewire or microcatheter navigation through the sinus may be complicated by vessel rupture. Alternatively, access to the cavernous sinus may be obtained through the facial vein or the superficial temporal vein. Direct operative cannulation of the superior ophthalmic vein is also an acceptable route to the cavernous sinus when other approaches have been exhausted. [34]

3. Imaging of DAVM

Recent advances in both computed tomography (CT) and magnetic resonance imaging (MRI) have significantly contributed to the initial diagnostic evaluation of patients with suspected DAVM. Because CT and MRI findings are nonspecific, however, the diagnosis can be delayed or missed. Routine conventional head CT is the first-line investigation of patients presenting with tinnitus, headache or other neurological symptoms. Its value is limited to identifying intracranial hemorrhage and edema due to venous congestion (area of low density). Focal or generalized atrophy of the brain, possibly accompanied by hydrocephalus, are nonspecific secondary findings that may be appreciated. Although not infrequently diagnostically equivocal, MRI is more helpful than CT because it can reveal dilated vessels, thrombosed venous structures, and prominent vascular enhancement particularly in patients with DAVM associated with CVD. The combination of prominent flow voids on the cortical surface and high-intensity lesions in the deep white matter on T2-weighted images secondary to venous hypertension/congestion is highly suggestive of a DAVM. Despite the presence of these secondary signs that suggest the presence of a DAVM, conventional MRI alone is generally unsuccessful in defining the exact site of fistulization. Any suspicious findings on CT/MRI should prompt catheter angiographic evaluation.

The advent of CT angiography (CTA) and magnetic resonance angiography (MRA) has provided more power to the noninvasive screening of patients with suspected DAVM. In addition to providing anatomic details, these modalities may be coupled with perfusion studies to evaluate the effect of a DAVM on regional blood flow.

CTA aids in the accurate diagnosis and characterization of DAVM by localizing the fistula and demonstrating the pattern of venous drainage and supplying arteries. Overlapping bone structures may make it difficult to demonstrate the detailed vascular pattern of DAVM especially for smaller lesions. The sensitivity of CTA for diagnosis of DAVM is reportedly lower than the sensitivity of MRA (15.4% versus 50%). [35] Lee et al [36] recently introduced a CTA algorithm for bone removal (hybrid CTA) that eliminates bone structures while preserving enhancing transosseous vascular structures. They found that the technique provides valuable information for treatment planning and carries a sensitivity of 93% and a specificity of 98%. In addition, recent studies have shown that 4D CTA with high spatial and temporal resolution are suitable for the diagnosis, classification, treatment planning, and follow-up imaging of DAVM. [37-38]

MRA may be performed using a three-dimensional time-of-flight (3D TOF) technique or MR digital subtraction angiography (MR DSA). [39-42] The presence of multiple high-intensity curvilinear or nodular structures adjacent to a sinus, in conjunction with high-intensity foci within the sinus is considered suspicious for a DAVM; however, the technique still suffers

http://dx.doi.org/10.5772/55219

from a high false positive rate, with as many as 14% of otherwise healthy patients incorrectly identified as possibly harboring a DAVM by 3D TOF MRA. Although the current spatial resolution of MR DSA is less than 3D TOF MRA, the benefit of MR DSA would be related to the temporal resolution of the technique and the ability to depict flow within cortical veins, particularly important in those patients with retrograde flow from a DAVM.

Despite the advances in both CTA and MRA, conventional digital subtraction angiography remains paramount in the diagnosis and pretreatment evaluation of intracranial DAVM.

The angiographic evaluation usually includes selective studies of the internal and external carotid arteries bilaterally as well as of both vertebral arteries when evaluating lesions of the posterior fossa or tentorium. The pretherapeutic examination must be tailored to the clinically suspected location of the fistula and must disclose the entire arterial supply, as well as any anastomoses between the supplying vessels and arterial distributions to the orbit, brain, or cranial nerves. This usually requires superselective arterial catheterization and angiography before the use of embolic materials. The venous anatomy must be studied with respect to the pattern of drainage from the fistula, and the adequacy of normal venous drainage of the brain must be assessed.

4. Therapeutic approaches to DAVM

Because many DAVM regress spontaneously or remain asymptomatic throughout the patient's life, it is crucial to weigh the risks of treatment against the natural history of these lesions. Management should be tailored to the type of lesion (location, classification, and angiographic features) and individual patient history (age, clinical presentation, and comorbidities) and may include relief of symptoms or complete occlusion of the DAVM. Although spontaneous resolution of clinical signs related to DAVM is not uncommon, most symptomatic lesions require some form of treatment. Treatment options include observation, carotid-jugular compression, transarterial embolization, transvenous embolization, open surgery and stereotactic radiosurgery. In the majority of patients, a multimodality approach with a combination of treatment offers the best chance for success.

Patients with Type I DAVM are at low risk of hemorrhage and should be managed conservatively unless they have disabling clinical symptoms like tinnitus or develop new neurological deficits or CVD at follow-up. Expectant follow-up of asymptomatic lesions should include serial MRI to detect changes in the DAVM anatomy. Angiographic follow-up should also be considered every few years especially for DAVM of the anterior cranial fossa or the tentorial incisura, which commonly develop CVD. Patients with symptomatic type II or III DAVM should be treated aggressively to minimize the risk of hemorrhage and NHND. The management of asymptomatic type II and III lesions should take into consideration the patient's age, treatment decision and risk of future hemorrhage. Intervention is often favored over observation because of the long-term risk to the patient and the dismal natural history of an intracranial hemorrhage.

Carotid-Jugular Compression. Patients with Borden type I transverse or sigmoid sinus DAVM or with fistulas of the cavernous sinus and otherwise normal ophthalmologic examinations may be treated conservatively with ipsilateral carotid or occipital artery compression. Intermittent manual compression of the carotid artery may be effective in eliminating DAVM involving the ipsilateral cavernous sinus in patients with mild findings and no evidence of carotid vascular disease or other contraindications to carotid compression. [21] The ipsilateral carotid artery is compressed, using the contralateral hand, for approximately 5 minutes every waking hour for 1 to 3 days. If this is tolerated, the compression time is increased to 10 to 15 minutes of compression per waking hour. The compression, if properly performed, produces concomitant partial obstruction of the ipsilateral carotid artery and jugular vein. This results in the transient reduction of arteriovenous shunting by decreasing arterial inflow while simultaneously increasing the outlet venous pressure, thereby promoting spontaneous thrombosis within the nidus. Nearly 30% of cavernous sinus and 25% of transverse/sigmoid sinus DAVM will thrombose with compression therapy. [43-44] Compression therapy is usually not recommended in patients with CVD.

Embolization. The development of improved superselective angiographic catheter systems and embolic agents has increased the role of interventional neuroradiology in the management of these lesions, both primarily and preoperatively. Two strategies, transvenous and transarterial have been employed and their appropriate selection depends on the location and complexity of the DAVM, its vascular features and the potential complications inherent to each technique. Treatment aims to completely occlude the arteriovenous fistula. If this is not an option, selective disconnection of the CVD is an acceptable option that is equally effective in reducing the risk of hemorrhage and NHND associated with DAVM. [45]

Transvenous embolization with metallic coils or detachable balloons has been advocated primarily for the treatment of DAVM involving the transverse, sigmoid or cavernous sinuses. The technique involves a transfemoral or intraoperative approach to the affected venous sinus following which coils, balloons or liquid embolic agents are deposited adjacent to the shunt. Several features are critical in appropriate patient selection for this method of treatment. (1) The segment of sinus to be occluded must be in proximity to the fistula and receive its entire venous drainage. (2) The sinus to be occluded should not be essential to the normal venous drainage of the brain. The cerebral venous drainage must be thoroughly evaluated before embolization to determine the alternate pathways for cerebral venous outflow and avoid potential venous infarction or hemorrhage. (3) The target sinus must be completely occluded throughout the involved segment to avoid diversion of fistulous flow into confluent cerebral veins and worsening of CVD. Such redirection of a high flow shunt into previously uninvolved low capacitance venous channels may precipitate an acute venous infarct or hemorrhage.

Levrier et al developed a novel way to treat DAVM that would preserve the venous sinus. [46] In ten patients including fistulas grade I-IV both with and without sinus stenosis, the researchers used a transvenous approach to angioplasty the involved sinus and then placed stents with high radial force to bridge the ostia of cortical veins draining into the sinus. Their follow-up at 7 months by conventional angiography revealed that four patients had complete DAVM occlusion and four had significantly reduced flow through the fistula. Two subjects refused repeat angiography. At two years, CTA confirmed stent patency in eight out of nine patients imaged. The safety and long-term efficacy of this technique, however, require further investigation.

Transvenous embolization is particularly useful for DAVM with multiple arterial feeders. Typically, involved arteries are small and torturous arterial feeders, which renders selective catheterization extremely challenging or hazardous. Ease of access to the fistulous site and the ability to obliterate the fistula in a single session are important advantages of this approach. Transvenous embolization is associated with a low complication rate and high rates of cure and complete occlusion of the fistula. [47-48] Transvenous embolization, however, is less suited for DAVM involving the superior sagittal sinus. It can also be associated with severe complications, including vessel rupture, sinus venous thrombosis, venous infarction, hemorrhage, and neurological deficits related to disruption of venous drainage. [49] Hemorrhage may be related to vessel injury or to the sacrifice of a dural sinus draining normal brain parenchyma. Additionally, transvenous embolization is rarely associated with the development of de novo DAVM at secondary intracranial sites following occlusion of the primary lesion. While the etiology of these secondary de novo fistulas is unclear, they may arise from angiogenesis induced by venous hypertension secondary to the occlusion of the major dural sinuses targeted by transvenous embolization.

Under some circumstances, transarterial embolization with liquid embolic agents offers advantages over a transvenous approach. Not infrequently, transvenous access to the DAVM is limited by venous sinus occlusion or high-grade stenoses preventing transvenous catheterization. Likewise, high-grade lesions emptying directly into remote small cerebral veins may be inaccessible to uncomplicated venous catheterization. As such, tentorial incisura and anterior cranial fossa DAVM, which frequently behave aggressively, may not be accessed transvenously. Transarterial delivery of a liquid embolic agent capable of permeating the vascular apparatus of the shunt provides the means for discrete definitive occlusion of the fistula site and reduces the likelihood for diversion of shunt flow into more dangerous alternate venous pathways while enabling closure of the fistula without necessarily sacrificing an entire venous conduit that may be critical to the drainage of normal brain parenchyma. Conversely, incomplete occlusion of the fistula by transarterial embolization is usually complicated by recruitment of new collateral vessels that are smaller, more tortuous and less amenable to embolization. Complex fistulas may require a multistaged approach combining transarterial and transvenous techniques to eliminate CVD and occlude the fistula.

Transarterial embolization may be effective in palliating disabling symptoms through occlusion of arterial feeders even without angiographic cure of the DAVM. Transarterial embolization also plays an important role in decreasing flow through DAVM before surgical intervention, transvenous obliteration, and radiosurgery. [50-51]

The transarterial approach requires selective catheterization of individual feeding vessels followed by superselective angiography to evaluate the vascular supply to the fistula, particularly with respect to potential anastomoses with the orbit or cerebral vasculature. It is important to understand that such anastomoses may not be demonstrable on the initial angiograms but may become manifest as progressive embolization produces alterations in flow within the target vascular territory.

Guidewire-directed microcatheters are typically employed in the catheterization of meningeal branches supplying such lesions. The embolic agents commonly used in transarterial embolization of DAVM are liquid cyanoacrylate (NBCA), Onyx, polyvinyl alcohol foam (PVA), or ethanol. Ideally, liquid embolic agents, delivered close to the shunt under wedged-microcatheter induced flow arrest, present the best opportunity for embolotherapeutic cure of the lesion as it enables permeation of the collateral complex supplying the fistula and its immediate venous receptacle thus permanently occluding the shunt. Such a degree of permeation is not possible using particulate agents that characteristically lodge within arterioles of the peri-fistula microcollateral network at a point proximal to the shunt. If not fully permeated, these microcollateral networks will then evolve and reestablish flow through the shunt complex.

Also, the particles degrade within days to weeks, resulting in high recurrence rates of the fistula and possibly in extensive shunting into leptomeningeal veins. Transarterial embolization with PVA is therefore used to relieve symptoms or in combination with other procedures such as radiation, surgery, or transvenous embolization. As with PVA, embolization with coils alone does not provide complete obliteration of DAVM. [52]

Nevertheless, PVA may find use in several situations. First, the initial use of PVA in embolizing the less favorable arterial supplies to a multi-pedicle fistula, may facilitate more complete subsequent embolization of the shunt with liquid embolic agents through a safer conduit. The embolization of competing inflows to the shunt with PVA allows the undiluted permeation of the fistula by the liquid embolic agent without fragmentation of the glue column. PVA may also be useful in reducing flow through low-velocity shunts, thereby facilitating thrombosis in these DAVM. This can be particularly applicable in managing low flow CSDAVM, and may be combined with manual compression in treating lesions also supplied by cavernous segment dural branches of the ipsilateral ICA.

In certain situations, partial embolization of dural fistulas may be performed in an attempt to alleviate disabling symptoms. For example, partial embolization of a cavernous sinus DAVM can reduce intraocular pressure in a patient suffering acute deterioration of visual acuity. Aggressive treatment in such cases may not be needed unless symptoms are particularly disabling or the DAVM is associated with CVD. Partial embolization may also be advocated in patients presenting with new-onset dementia or in those patients with severe tinnitus. Lastly, PVA and liquid embolic agents are used in the preoperative devascularization of dural fistulas prior to surgical excision. In this situation, particulate embolic agents, because of their low morbidity, are generally preferred and should be applied 1 to 2 days before surgery.

NBCA has been widely utilized for transarterial embolization of DAVM with fairly good results. Guedin et al [53] treated 43 patients with Borden Type II or III DAVM using NBCA and reported complete obliteration of the fistula in 34 patients (79%) and occlusion of CVD in all remaining cases. There was no treatment-related mortality or permanent morbidity in the series. Interestingly, they reported post-embolization secondary thrombosis in 5 patients in whom residual flow was noted on the immediate post-treatment angiograms. In a recent large study by Kim et al [54] that included 121 DAVM treated with transarterial glue embolization, immediate cure was achieved in 14.0% of lesions, and progressive complete thrombosis of the residual shunt at follow-up in 15.7% of lesions. Surgical CVD disconnection or transvenous coil embolization was necessary for clinically important residual shunts in as many as 45.2% of all cases. Procedural complications were seen in 7.8% of patients in the series.

However, use of NBCA has some disadvantages. It is an adhesive agent that undergoes rapid polymerization at contact with blood, which may increase the risk of microcatheter retention or avulsion of the feeding artery upon removal of the microcatheter. The injection must be performed quickly and continuously, which may diminish the precision of injection and result in suboptimal penetration into the fistulous site. Use of a wedged microcatheter technique with low-concentration glue may maximize glue penetration into the venous drainage route (Figure 1).

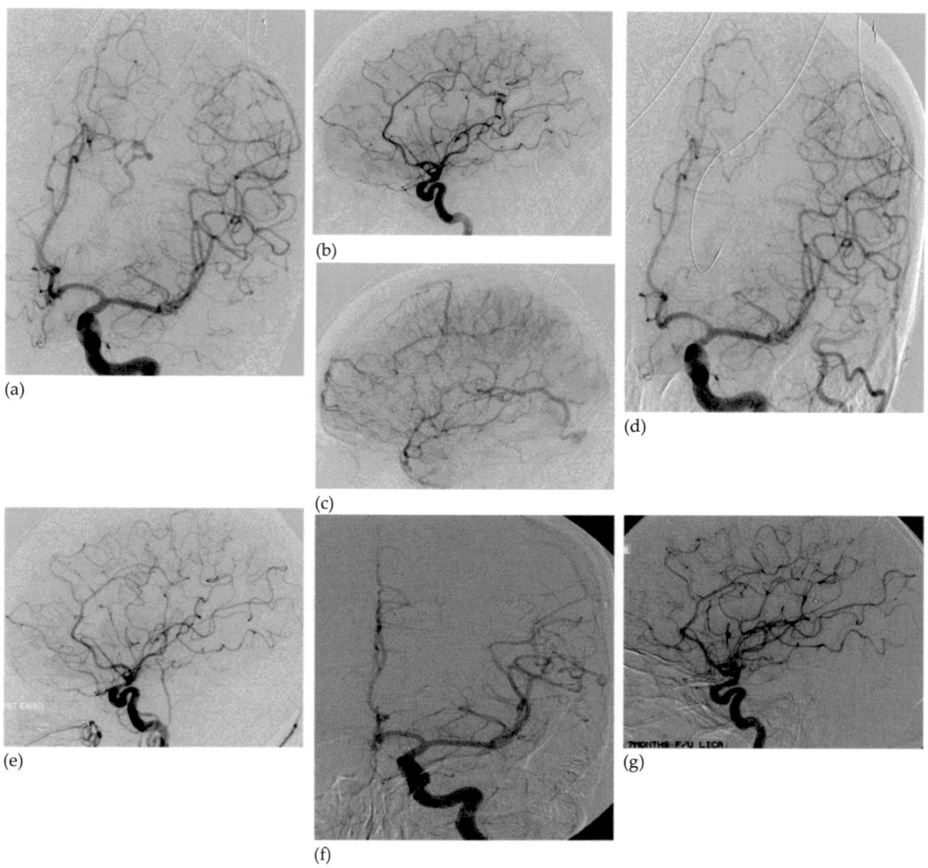

Figure 1. Frontal (A) and lateral (B, C) views of digital subtraction angiography (DSA) in a 50-year-old woman who sustained an intraventricular hemorrhage showing a DAVM fed by posterior branches of the pericallosal artery and draining into the straight sinus. Frontal (D) and lateral (E) views of DSA following embolization with 0.4 mL of NBCA 40% showing complete occlusion of the fistula. Frontal (F) and lateral (G) views of follow-up DSA 7 months later showing durable occlusion of the DAVM.

Recently, the introduction of Onyx has added an important element to the endovascular armamentarium and improved the endovascular treatment of DAVM. Onyx is comprised of ethylene vinyl alcohol copolymer dissolved in DMSO (dimethyl sulfoxide), and suspended micronized tantalum powder to provide contrast for visualization under fluoroscopy. Onyx offers several advantages over NBCA, which allow for safer and more efficient treatment of DAVM. Due to its lava-like flow pattern and its nonadhesive nature, Onyx facilitates longer, slower, and more controlled injections with better penetration of the fistula. It also allows embolization of a substantial portion of the lesion from a single pedicle injection because the agent can efficiently penetrate the depths of the fistulous connection and then flow into adjacent arterial feeders, thereby obviating the need for multiple embolizations. The interventionalist can even discontinue Onyx injection for angiographic assessment of the embolization and evaluation of collateral and en passage feeders that may become evident during the course of embolization. Additionally, Onyx is less adherent to the microcatheter than NBCA with possibly a lower risk of catheter retention and arterial rupture. The middle meningeal artery provides an excellent route for Onyx injection with particularly high curative rates according to several reports. [55-57] The middle meningeal artery is easy to catheterize and its branches are anchored to the dura and calvarium, which facilitates removal of the microcatheter and minimizes the risk of arterial avulsion.

Onyx has some disadvantages compared to NBCA, namely an increase in fluoroscopy time, procedure time, and procedure cost. Cranial nerve injury and DMSO-induced angiotoxicity are additional disadvantages of Onyx. There is also a risk of distal embolization of the embolic material into the venous system and the pulmonary circulation.

Several investigators have reported remarkably high cure rates with this embolic agent, with a high proportion of treatments completed in a single session. [49] Cognard et al enrolled 30 patients in a prospective trial: ten were graded type II, eight type III and twelve type IV fistulas. [55] They reported complete anatomic cure in 24/30 patients with only two complications, including a temporary cranial nerve palsy and post-procedure hemorrhage secondary to venous outlet thrombosis. Lv et al report their experience with 40 patients suffering from DAVM. [27, 58] They report a complete occlusion rate of 25/40 or 62.3%. Nine patients suffered complications including reflexive bradyarrhythmia in 3 patients, hemifacial hypoesthesia in 3, hemifacial palsy in 2, posterior infarction in 2, jaw pain in 1, hallucinations in 1, Onyx migration in 1 and retention of a microcatheter tip in 1. Abud et al [59] treated 44 DAVM with Onyx and achieved occlusion of the shunt in all but 9 patients, 5 of whom were successfully treated by complimentary transvenous embolization with coils and Onyx. In as many as 81% of cases, a cure was obtained in a single session. Six complications were observed including 4 cranial nerve injuries and 2 cases of venous thrombosis post-embolization. In a series of 29 DAVM treated with Onyx embolization, mostly through a transarterial approach, Stiefel et al [56] achieved an angiographic cure in 72% of all lesions, with complications occurring in 9.7% of cases and leading into permanent morbidity in only 2.4%. We have recently reviewed our experience in 39 patients with DAVM treated between 2001 and 2009 at Jefferson Hospital for Neuroscience. We found no major procedure-related complications in the series and achieved an obliteration rate of 75% with elimination of CVD in up to 85% of patients with Onyx embolization (Figure 2-3).

http://dx.doi.org/10.5772/55219

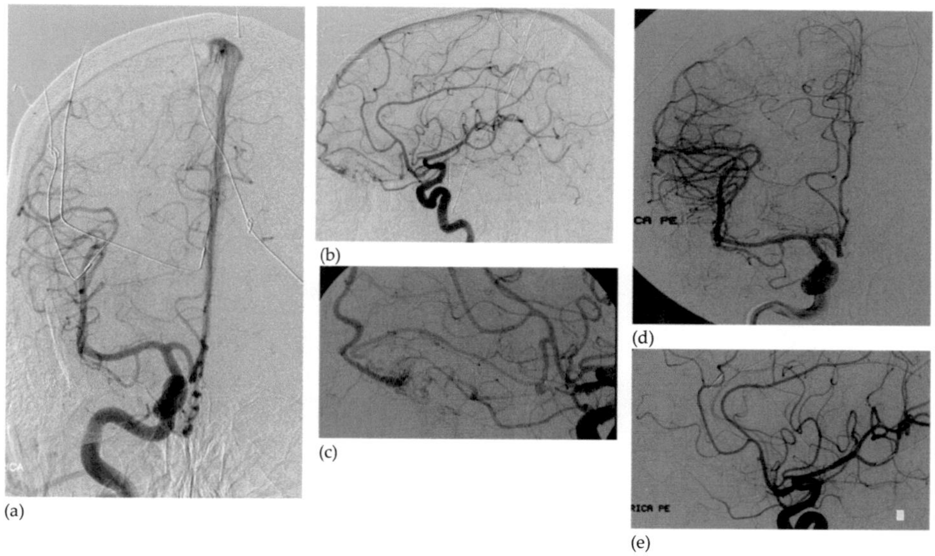

Figure 2. Frontal (A) and lateral (B) views of digital subtraction angiography (DSA) in a 66-year-old woman who sustained a subarachnoid hemorrhage showing an ethmoidal DAVM, fed by the ophthalmic artery and anterior ethmoidal branches, as well as an orbito-frontal branch of the anterior cerebral artery. A small 1 mm aneurysm is seen on the orbito-frontal feeding vessel. The DAVM demonstrates CVD with a draining vein entering the anterior 1/3 of the superior sagittal sinus. (C) Superselective injection through the orbito-frontal pedicle showing the aneurysm and the fistula. The aneurysm and the fistula were embolized with 0.1 ml of Onyx through the orbito-frontal pedicle. Frontal (D) and lateral (E) views of DSA after embolization showing obliteration of the aneurysm and the fistula.

A few investigators have used Onyx in a transvenous approach to carotid-cavernous fistulas. After an unsuccessful embolization of a C-C fistula using detachable coils and liquid adhesion agents, Arat et al successfully completed the embolization by injecting Onyx into the cavernous sinus forming a cast of the structure. [60-61] Similarly, He et al report their experience in 6 patients using a combination of detachable coils and Onyx via a transvenous approach. [62] Four of the six cases were completely embolized in one attempt, whereas the other two required staged procedures. In these latter two cases the patient suffered minor transient cranial nerve palsies. Suzuki et al report equally good results in three patients with spontaneous C-C fistulas. [63] In all these studies patients experienced rapid relief of their neuro-ophthalmologic symptoms. El Hammady et al [64] treated 12 patients with C-C fistulas using Onyx, 8 through a transvenous route and 4 through a transarterial route. All lesions in their series were obliterated in a single session with resolution of presenting symptoms in 100% of patients by 2 months. Cranial neuropathies, however, were noted in 3 patients likely from post-embolization cavernous sinus thrombosis and swelling or from cranial nerve ischemia/infarction from deep penetration of Onyx. We have recently reported on Onyx embolization of C-C fistulas through a surgical cannulation of the superior ophthalmic vein in a series of 10 patients. [34] We achieved complete obliteration of the fistula in 8 patients and a significant reduction in fistulous flow in 2 patients, with no procedural complications.

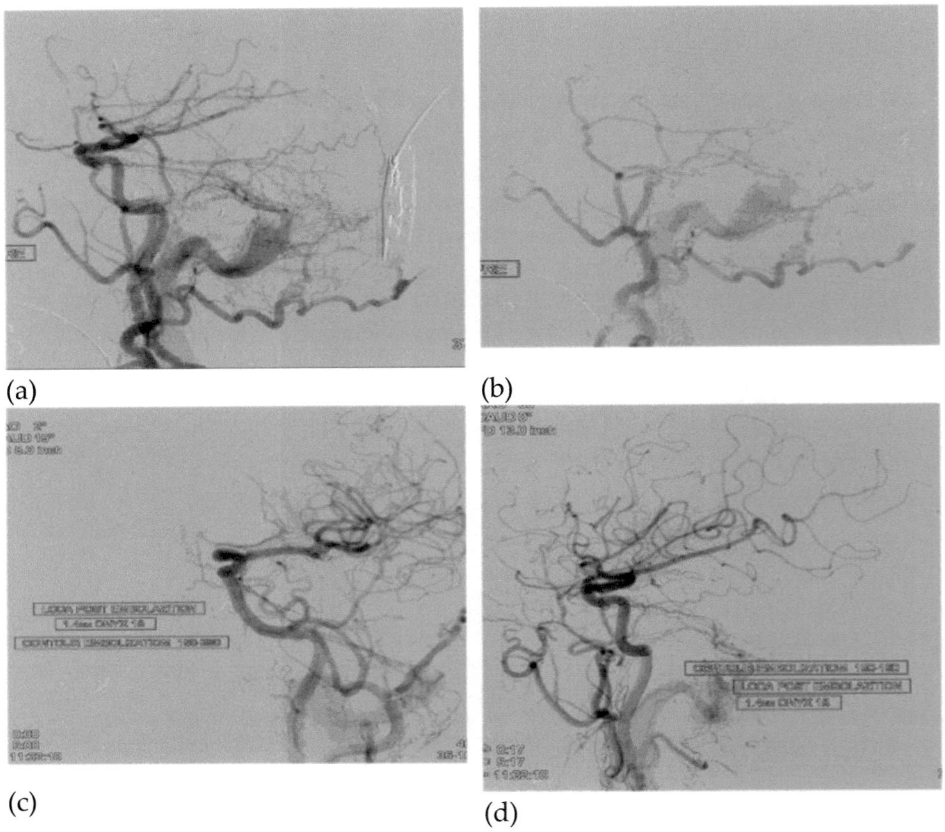

Figure 3. Lateral views of left common carotid artery (A) and left external carotid artery (B) injections of DSA in a 65-year-old woman with severe disabling tinnitus showing a tentorial DAVM draining into the transverse-sigmoid junction with no evidence of CVD. Feeding vessels arise from the superficial temporal artery, middle meningeal artery, occipital artery, and posterior auricular artery. The fistula was treated by embolization with Onyx and PVA through the left occipital artery, left middle meningeal branches, left posterior auricular artery, and superficial temporal arteries. Frontal (C) and lateral (D) views of DSA after embolization showing significant reduction in flow through the fistula.

5. The role of surgery

With the advent of Onyx, most lesions can now be successfully managed with endovascular therapy. However, surgical treatment of DAVM may still be necessary when endovascular options have failed. Surgery consists of disconnection of draining veins, disconnection of arterial feeders, resection/packing of the dural sinus, and/or direct puncture and embolization of large varices or meningeal arteries. Hoh et al [65] described a technique whereby the draining vein is clipped close to the fistula with extensive dural coagulation.

DAVM of the anterior cranial fossa and the superior sagittal sinus are more suitable for surgical treatment than other types of DAVM. Transarterial embolization plays an important role in decreasing flow through the DAVM prior to surgical intervention and facilitates operative exposure of the involved segment of the dural sinuses, thus affecting the quality and completeness of surgical excision.

6. The role of stereotactic radiosurgery

Stereotactic radiosurgery is an acceptable option for DAVM not amenable to surgical or endovascular therapies. It is best suited for benign lesions without CVD (type I) and for low-flow cavernous DAVM (which typically do not have CVD). Radiosurgery induces thrombogenic obliteration of DAVM with a latency period of up to two years. This treatment modality is therefore not suitable for DAVM with CVD because such lesions have a malignant natural history and require rapid and definitive treatment via surgical or endovascular means. A recent review of 14 studies found that stereotactic radiosurgery with or without adjunctive embolization results in DAVM obliteration in 71% of cases and post-treatment hemorrhage in 1.6% of cases (4.8% of lesions with CVD). [66] Despite these promising results, experience with radiosurgery in DAVM treatment remains limited and the efficacy of the technique requires more investigation in large prospective studies. Meanwhile, stereotactic radiosurgery should be reserved for lesions that are not amenable to surgical or endovascular interventions.

7. Conclusion

Recent advances in endovascular therapies and studies of the anatomical and functional properties of DAVM led to a rapid evolution in their diagnosis and management. Onyx embolization through transarterial or transvenous approaches has emerged as safe and highly efficient treatment for even the most complex lesions. However, the decision of which approach and embolic agent to use for treatment of a DAVM must be tailored to each individual case, recognizing that the most effective approach for permanent DAVM treatment, particularly in high-flow shunts, may require a combination of approaches and embolic agents. Treatment of DAVM should be entrusted to a multidisciplinary team with ample expertise in the management of these often challenging lesions.

Author details

Nohra Chalouhi, Pascal Jabbour, Aaron S. Dumont, L. Fernando Gonzalez,
Robert Rosenwasser and Stavropoula Tjoumakaris*

*Address all correspondence to: stavropoula.tjoumakaris@jefferson.edu

Department of Neurosurgery, Thomas Jefferson University and Jefferson Hospital for Neuroscience, Philadelphia, Pennsylvania, USA

References

[1] Narayanan, S. Endovascular management of intracranial dural arteriovenous fistulas. Neurol Clin. (2010). Nov;, 28(4), 899-911.

[2] Mcconnell, K. A, Tjoumakaris, S. I, Allen, J, Shapiro, M, Bescke, T, Jabbour, P. M, et al. Neuroendovascular management of dural arteriovenous malformations. Neurosurg Clin N Am. (2009). Oct;, 20(4), 431-9.

[3] Tsai, L. K, Jeng, J. S, Liu, H. M, Wang, H. J, & Yip, P. K. Intracranial dural arteriovenous fistulas with or without cerebral sinus thrombosis: analysis of 69 patients. J Neurol Neurosurg Psychiatry. (2004). Nov;, 75(11), 1639-41.

[4] Gerlach, R, Yahya, H, Rohde, S, Bohm, M, Berkefeld, J, Scharrer, I, et al. Increased incidence of thrombophilic abnormalities in patients with cranial dural arteriovenous fistulae. Neurol Res. (2003). Oct;, 25(7), 745-8.

[5] Surgical neuroangiographyClinical and endovascular treatment...., 2

[6] Lv, X, Jiang, C, Li, Y, Liu, L, Liu, J, & Wu, Z. Transverse-sigmoid sinus dural arteriovenous fistulae. World Neurosurg. (2010). Aug-Sep;74(2-3):297-305.

[7] Borden, J. A, Wu, J. K, & Shucart, W. A. A proposed classification for spinal and cranial dural arteriovenous fistulous malformations and implications for treatment. J Neurosurg. (1995). Feb;, 82(2), 166-79.

[8] Cognard, C, Gobin, Y. P, Pierot, L, Bailly, A. L, Houdart, E, Casasco, A, et al. Cerebral dural arteriovenous fistulas: clinical and angiographic correlation with a revised classification of venous drainage. Radiology. (1995). Mar;, 194(3), 671-80.

[9] Davies, M. A. TerBrugge K, Willinsky R, Coyne T, Saleh J, Wallace MC. The validity of classification for the clinical presentation of intracranial dural arteriovenous fistulas. J Neurosurg. (1996). Nov;, 85(5), 830-7.

[10] Duffau, H, Lopes, M, Janosevic, V, Sichez, J. P, Faillot, T, Capelle, L, et al. Early rebleeding from intracranial dural arteriovenous fistulas: report of 20 cases and review of the literature. J Neurosurg. (1999). Jan;, 90(1), 78-84.

[11] Satomi, J, Van Dijk, J. M, Terbrugge, K. G, Willinsky, R. A, & Wallace, M. C. Benign cranial dural arteriovenous fistulas: outcome of conservative management based on the natural history of the lesion. J Neurosurg. (2002). Oct;, 97(4), 767-70.

[12] Shah, M. N, Botros, J. A, Pilgram, T. K, Moran, C. J, & Cross, D. T. rd, Chicoine MR, et al. Borden-Shucart Type I dural arteriovenous fistulas: clinical course including risk of conversion to higher-grade fistulas. J Neurosurg. (2012). Sep;, 117(3), 539-45.

[13] Davies, M. A, & Saleh, J. Ter Brugge K, Willinsky R, Wallace MC. The natural history and management of intracranial dural arteriovenous fistulae. Part 1: benign lesions. Interv Neuroradiol. (1997). Dec 20;, 3(4), 295-302.

[14] Davies, M. A. Ter Brugge K, Willinsky R, Wallace MC. The natural history and management of intracranial dural arteriovenous fistulae. Part 2: aggressive lesions. Interv Neuroradiol. (1997). Dec 20;, 3(4), 303-11.

[15] Van Dijk, J. M. terBrugge KG, Willinsky RA, Wallace MC. Clinical course of cranial dural arteriovenous fistulas with long-term persistent cortical venous reflux. Stroke. (2002). May;, 33(5), 1233-6.

[16] Soderman, M, Pavic, L, Edner, G, Holmin, S, & Andersson, T. Natural history of dural arteriovenous shunts. Stroke. (2008). Jun;, 39(6), 1735-9.

[17] Strom, R. G, Botros, J. A, Refai, D, Moran, C. J, & Cross, D. T. rd, Chicoine MR, et al. Cranial dural arteriovenous fistulae: asymptomatic cortical venous drainage portends less aggressive clinical course. Neurosurgery. (2009). Feb;discussion 7-8., 64(2), 241-7.

[18] Zipfel, G. J, Shah, M. N, Refai, D, & Dacey, R. G. Jr., Derdeyn CP. Cranial dural arteriovenous fistulas: modification of angiographic classification scales based on new natural history data. Neurosurg Focus. (2009). May;26(5):E14.

[19] Dural arteriovenous shunts: a new classification of craniospinal epidural venous anatomical bases and clinical correlations. (2008).

[20] Dural arteriovenous fistula: diagnosistreatment, and outcomes, ((2009).

[21] Youmans Neurological Surgery Edition: Text with Continually Updated Online. (2003).

[22] Endovascular treatment of pure spontaneous dural vascular malformationsReview of 23 cases studied and treated between May 1980 and October 1983], ((1984).

[23] Nakahara, Y, Ogata, A, Takase, Y, Maeda, K, Okamoto, H, Matsushima, T, et al. Treatment of dural arteriovenous fistula presenting as typical symptoms of hydrocephalus caused by venous congestion: case report. Neurol Med Chir (Tokyo). (2011). , 51(3), 229-32.

[24] Hydrocephalus in unruptured brain arteriovenous malformations: pathomechanical considerationstherapeutic implications, and clinical course, ((2009).

[25] Bulters, D. O, Mathad, N, Culliford, D, Millar, J, & Sparrow, O. C. The natural history of cranial dural arteriovenous fistulae with cortical venous reflux--the significance of venous ectasia. Neurosurgery. (2012). Feb;discussion 8-9., 70(2), 312-8.

[26] [Diagnosis and treatment of tentorial dural arteriovenous fistulae]. (2005).

[27] Endovascular treatment of anterior cranial fossa dural arteriovenous fistula. (2008).

[28] Agid, R, Terbrugge, K, Rodesch, G, Andersson, T, & Soderman, M. Management strategies for anterior cranial fossa (ethmoidal) dural arteriovenous fistulas with an emphasis on endovascular treatment. J Neurosurg. (2009). Jan;, 110(1), 79-84.

[29] Kiyosue, H, Hori, Y, Okahara, M, Tanoue, S, Sagara, Y, Matsumoto, S, et al. Treatment of intracranial dural arteriovenous fistulas: current strategies based on location and hemodynamics, and alternative techniques of transcatheter embolization. Radiographics. (2004). Nov-Dec;, 24(6), 1637-53.

[30] Assessment of dural arteriovenous fistulas of the cavernous sinuses on 3D dynamic MR angiography. (2008).

[31] Coil embolization of cavernous sinus in patients with direct and dural arteriovenous fistula. (2009).

[32] Cavernous sinus dural arteriovenous malformations: patterns of venous drainage are related to clinical signs and symptoms. (2002).

[33] Bilateral orbital signs predict cortical venous drainage in cavernous sinus dural AVMs. (2002).

[34] Chalouhi, N, Dumont, A. S, Tjoumakaris, S, Gonzalez, L. F, Bilyk, J. R, Randazzo, C, et al. The superior ophthalmic vein approach for the treatment of carotid-cavernous fistulas: a novel technique using Onyx. Neurosurg Focus. (2012). May;32(5):E13.

[35] Cohen, S. D, Goins, J. L, Butler, S. G, Morris, P. P, & Browne, J. D. Dural arteriovenous fistula: diagnosis, treatment, and outcomes. Laryngoscope. (2009). Feb;, 119(2), 293-7.

[36] Lee, C. W, Huang, A, Wang, Y. H, Yang, C. Y, Chen, Y. F, & Liu, H. M. Intracranial dural arteriovenous fistulas: diagnosis and evaluation with 64-detector row CT angiography. Radiology. (2010). Jul;, 256(1), 219-28.

[37] Brouwer, P. A, Bosman, T, Van Walderveen, M. A, Krings, T, Leroux, A. A, & Willems, P. W. Dynamic 320-section CT angiography in cranial arteriovenous shunting lesions. AJNR Am J Neuroradiol. (2010). Apr;, 31(4), 767-70.

[38] Siebert, E, Bohner, G, Dewey, M, Masuhr, F, Hoffmann, K. T, Mews, J, et al. slice CT neuroimaging: initial clinical experience and image quality evaluation. Br J Radiol. (2009). Jul;, 82(979), 561-70.

[39] Assessment of 3D-TOF-MRA at 3Tesla in the characterization of the angioarchitecture of cerebral arteriovenous malformations: a preliminary study, ((2007).

[40] Contrast-enhanced, M. R. D angiography in the assessment of brain AVMs, ((2006).

[41] MR angiography fusion technique for treatment planning of intracranial arteriovenous malformations, (2006).

[42] MR angiography of dural arteriovenous fistulas: diagnosis and follow-up after treatment using a time-resolved 3D contrast-enhanced technique, (2007).

[43] Halbach, V. V, Higashida, R. T, Hieshima, G. B, Reicher, M, Norman, D, & Newton, T. H. Dural fistulas involving the cavernous sinus: results of treatment in 30 patients. Radiology. (1987). May;, 163(2), 437-42.

[44] Halbach, V. V, Higashida, R. T, Hieshima, G. B, Goto, K, Norman, D, & Newton, T. H. Dural fistulas involving the transverse and sigmoid sinuses: results of treatment in 28 patients. Radiology. (1987). May;, 163(2), 443-7.

[45] Mironov, A. Selective transvenous embolization of dural fistulas without occlusion of the dural sinus. AJNR Am J Neuroradiol. (1998). Feb;, 19(2), 389-91.

[46] Use of a self-expanding stent with balloon angioplasty in the treatment of dural arteriovenous fistulas involving the transverse and/or sigmoid sinus: functional and neuroimaging-based outcome in 10 patients. (2006).

[47] Yoshida, K, Melake, M, Oishi, H, Yamamoto, M, & Arai, H. Transvenous embolization of dural carotid cavernous fistulas: a series of 44 consecutive patients. AJNR Am J Neuroradiol. (2010). Apr;, 31(4), 651-5.

[48] Klisch, J, Huppertz, H. J, Spetzger, U, Hetzel, A, Seeger, W, & Schumacher, M. Transvenous treatment of carotid cavernous and dural arteriovenous fistulae: results for 31 patients and review of the literature. Neurosurgery. (2003). Oct;discussion 56-7., 53(4), 836-56.

[49] Gandhi, D, Chen, J, Pearl, M, Huang, J, Gemmete, J. J, & Kathuria, S. Intracranial dural arteriovenous fistulas: classification, imaging findings, and treatment. AJNR Am J Neuroradiol. (2012). Jun;, 33(6), 1007-13.

[50] Friedman, J. A, Pollock, B. E, Nichols, D. A, Gorman, D. A, Foote, R. L, & Stafford, S. L. Results of combined stereotactic radiosurgery and transarterial embolization for dural arteriovenous fistulas of the transverse and sigmoid sinuses. J Neurosurg. (2001). Jun;, 94(6), 886-91.

[51] Goto, K, Sidipratomo, P, Ogata, N, Inoue, T, & Matsuno, H. Combining endovascular and neurosurgical treatments of high-risk dural arteriovenous fistulas in the lateral sinus and the confluence of the sinuses. J Neurosurg. (1999). Feb;, 90(2), 289-99.

[52] Cognard, C, Houdart, E, Casasco, A, Gabrillargues, J, Chiras, J, & Merland, J. J. Long-term changes in intracranial dural arteriovenous fistulae leading to worsening in the type of venous drainage. Neuroradiology. (1997). Jan;, 39(1), 59-66.

[53] Guedin, P, Gaillard, S, Boulin, A, Condette-auliac, S, Bourdain, F, Guieu, S, et al. Therapeutic management of intracranial dural arteriovenous shunts with leptomeningeal venous drainage: report of 53 consecutive patients with emphasis on transarterial embolization with acrylic glue. J Neurosurg. (2010). Mar;, 112(3), 603-10.

[54] Kim, D. J, Willinsky, R. A, Krings, T, Agid, R, & Terbrugge, K. Intracranial dural arteriovenous shunts: transarterial glue embolization--experience in 115 consecutive patients. Radiology. (2011). Feb;, 258(2), 554-61.

[55] Endovascular treatment of intracranial dural arteriovenous fistulas with cortical venous drainage: new management using Onyx. (2008).

[56] Stiefel, M. F, Albuquerque, F. C, Park, M. S, Dashti, S. R, & Mcdougall, C. G. Endovascular treatment of intracranial dural arteriovenous fistulae using Onyx: a case series. Neurosurgery. (2009). Dec;65(6 Suppl):discussion 9-40., 132-9.

[57] Hu, Y. C, Newman, C. B, Dashti, S. R, Albuquerque, F. C, & Mcdougall, C. G. Cranial dural arteriovenous fistula: transarterial Onyx embolization experience and technical nuances. J Neurointerv Surg. (2011). Mar;, 3(1), 5-13.

[58] Endovascular treatment of brain arteriovenous fistulas. (2009).

[59] Abud, T. G, Nguyen, A, Saint-maurice, J. P, Abud, D. G, Bresson, D, Chiumarulo, L, et al. The use of Onyx in different types of intracranial dural arteriovenous fistula. AJNR Am J Neuroradiol. (2011). Dec;, 32(11), 2185-91.

[60] Embolization of high-flow craniofacial vascular malformations with onyx. (2007).

[61] Treatment of a superior sagittal sinus dural arteriovenous fistula with Onyx: technical case report. (2006).

[62] Transvenous embolization with a combination of detachable coils and Onyx for a complicated cavernous dural arteriovenous fistula. (2008).

[63] Transvenous treatment of spontaneous dural carotid-cavernous fistulas using a combination of detachable coils and Onyx. (2006).

[64] Elhammady, M. S, Wolfe, S. Q, Farhat, H, Moftakhar, R, & Aziz-sultan, M. A. Onyx embolization of carotid-cavernous fistulas. J Neurosurg. (2010). Mar;, 112(3), 589-94.

[65] Hoh, B. L, Choudhri, T. F, & Connolly, E. S. Jr., Solomon RA. Surgical management of high-grade intracranial dural arteriovenous fistulas: leptomeningeal venous disruption without nidus excision. Neurosurgery. (1998). Apr;discussion-5., 42(4), 796-804.

[66] Gross, B. A, Ropper, A. E, Popp, A. J, & Du, R. Stereotactic radiosurgery for cerebral dural arteriovenous fistulas. Neurosurg Focus. (2012). May;32(5):E18.

Chapter 2

Percutaneous Transvenous Embolization of Intracranial Dural Arteriovenous Fistulas with Detachable Coils and/or in Combination with Onyx

Xianli Lv, Youxiang Li and Chuhan Jiang

Additional information is available at the end of the chapter

http://dx.doi.org/10.5772/56732

1. Introduction

Intracranial dural arteriovenous fistulas (DAVFs) represent 10 to 15% of intracranial arteriovenous malformation. [1-3] Published classifications of DAVFs (e.g., Cognard's classification) are based on the pattern of drainage, for estimation of bleeding risks. [4] Venous drainage patterns allow classification of DAVFs into five types as follows: Type I, located in the main sinus, with anterograde flow; Type II, located in the main sinus, with reflux into the sinus (Type IIa), cortical veins (Type IIb), or both (Type IIa+b); Type III, with direct cortical venous drainage without venous ectasia; Type IV, with direct cortical venous drainage with venous ectasia; Type V, with spinal venous drainage (Table1). Depending on the DAVFs location and the venous drainage, clinical presentations range from asymptomatic to symptomatic [5-11], with pulse-synchronous bruit, headaches, neurological deficits, venous hypertensive encephalopathy with dementia, or intracranial hemorrhage resulting from venous hypertension.

The decision to treat is based on the venous drainage pattern, the natural history of the lesion, the severity of presenting symptoms, the patient's general condition, angiographic features, the location of the DAVF, and the morbidity and mortality rates of the procedure being considered. The goals of treatment are the prevention of risks and the elimination of symptoms caused by the arteriovenous shunt. Because of the bleeding risk, intracranial DAVFs with retrograde cortical drainage often require an anatomic cure. They can be treated with different modalities, such as endovascular procedures with transvenous and transarterial [2, 3, 5, 11-36], surgery [6-8, 35, 37-43], gamma knife surgery [31, 44-47], or combinations of the three [7, 24, 48-50]; in selected cases, the lesions can be treated conservatively [20].

2. Transvenous technique

The embolization of DAVFs is performed under general anesthesia, preferably under supervision of an experienced neuroanesthesiologist. Transvenous catheterizations and embolizations are often lengthy procedures (2–4 h), during which the typically elderly patients would have difficulties remaining still on an angiographic table. General anesthesia with endotracheal intubation is therefore widely used in most centers in the world, as it also allows for safer monitoring and easier management in cases of intraprocedural complications such as rupture and hemorrhage. Bilateral selective internal carotid artery (ICA) and external carotid artery (ECA) angiography and vertebral artery (VA) angiography were performed for all patients, for assessment of the feeding arteries, the fistula sites and the venous drainage. The arteriovenous shunts were approached via the venous route. We first placed 6-French sheaths in the femoral artery and vein. A 5-French catheter in the carotid artery allowed observation of the shunt, acquisition of roadmaps, and angiographic monitoring of the procedure. A second 5-French catheter was placed in the jugular vein. A microcatheter (Marathon/Echelon, MTI-EV3, Irvine, CA, USA) was navigated coaxially via different venous approaches. The microguiderwire (Mirage/Silverspeed10, MTI-EV3, Irvine, CA, USA; Transend0.014, Boston Scientific, USA) was then carefully introduced and advanced to the fistula portion, followed by the microcatheter. Subsequently, the draining vein or sinus was packed using detachable platinum coils or a combination with Onyx, using real-time digital subtraction fluoroscopic mapping.

3. Case reports (Figs.1-8)

3.1. Case report I: Ethmoidal DAVF (Fig.1)

A 48-year-old man with a DAVF of the anterior ranial fossa supplied by branches of the anterior ethmoidal arteries, the septal branches of the sphenopalatine and the middle meningeal arteries with venous drainage via dilated frontopolar veins to the superior sagittal sinus. A guide catheter was inserted into the jugular vein transfemorally and a microcatheter (Echelon10, MTI-ev3, Irvine, CA) was navigated over a guidewire (Silverspeed, MTI-EV3, Irvine, CA, USA) to the frontal part of the superior sagittal sinus. The microcatheter was gently advanced into the primary draining vein. Once the tip of the microcatheter had reached the fistula point, embolization was performed with detachable platinum coils until transarterial angiography showed occlusion of the DAVF (Fig. 1).

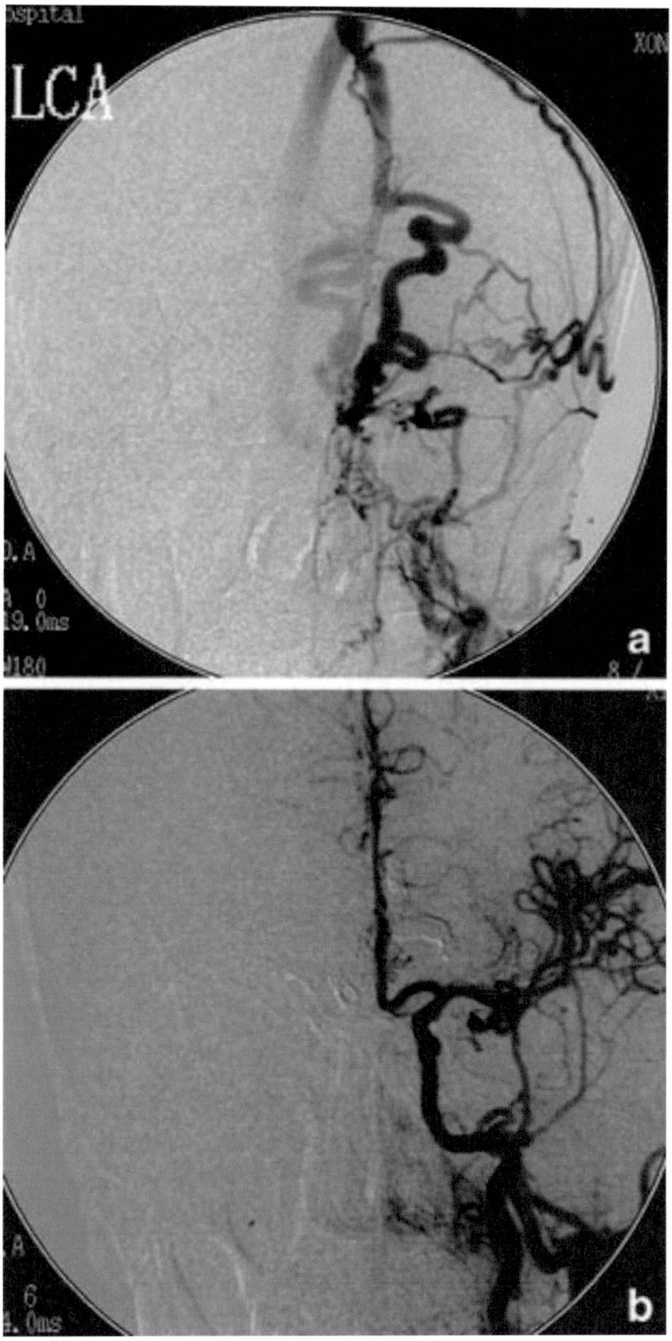

Figure 1. a, Left ECA angiogram shows the fistula fed by the left sphenopalatine artery and the left middle meningeal artery. b, Frontal angiogram following injection of the left common carotid artery (CCA) with coils placed in bilateral dilated frontopolar veins shows occlusion of the fistula.

3.2. Case report II:Cavernous DAVF (IPS) (Fig.2)

A 54-year-old man presented with blepharoptosis, diplopia and chemosis for 2 months. Cerebral angiograms were obtained and showed a DAVF principally fed by the left meningohypophyseal trunk with additional small branches of the right ICA. Venous outflow empted into the left inferior petroal sinus (IPS) and the left superior ophthalmic vein (SOV). Recommendation was made for transvenous embolization of this lesion. Under general anesthesia, catheterization was performed via transfemoral approach using standard coaxial techniques. Systemic heparinization was achieved during the procedures with heparin 3000U bolus followed by 1000U of heparin every hour. A 5-French diagnostic catheter with continuous heparized flush was positioned in the left ICA for selective control angiograms. The late venous phase of the left ICA angiogram revealed the IPS on this side. Therefore, this IPS was chosen for endovascular approach. A 5-F guiding catheter was placed and, using road mapping technique and fluoroscopic guidance, a microcatheter (Echelon14, MTI-EV3, Irvine, CA, USA) was advanced over a guidwire (Transend0.014, Boston Scientific) into the left IPS up to the left cavernous sinus (CS). Three hydrocoils (two 5×12, one 6×15; MicroPlex) were packed first to reduce the venous outflow towards the SOV. Then, under biplane roadmapping, the catheter was slowly flushed with 0.25ml of DMSO over 40 seconds and this was followed by injection of Onyx (MTI-EV3, Irvine, CA, USA). After 2.3ml of Onyx-34 was injected into the cavernous sinus, we attempted to inject Onyx-18. In the meantime caution was exerted to avoid inadvertent embolization of the left ICA during the slow injection of Onyx. Patency of the left ICA was checked frequently during the intermittent injection of the embolic material. The amount of injected Onyx-18 was 2.6ml. The procedure was completed as soon as a control angiogram revealed complete occlusion of the DAVF. The patient's chemosis improved within the next day, but blepharotosis and diplopia were not improved. The patient was discharged on the postprocedure day 3.

3.3. Case report III :Cavernous DAVF (Cross-over approach via IPS) (Fig.3)

A 44-year-old woman demonstrated right proptosis and VIth cranial nerve palsy and excessive pulsatile bruits. Cerebral angiography revealed a DAVF of the right CS.Angiography of the right CCA demonstrated persistent filling of the left IPS (Figure 1A). Therefore, a transvenous approach was chosen. The microcatheter was navigated through the left IPS and the intercavernous sinus to the right CS (Figure 1C).The right CS was occluded with 28 standard coils (Figure 1D, E). However, the pulsatile tinnitus was still persistent at six-month follow-up study. Control angiography demonstrated recurrence of the fistula (Figure 1F) and the same procedure was performed (Figure 1G). The residual fistula was occluded completely by another six standard coils (Figure 1H).

3.4. Case report IV:Cavernous DAVF (FV-SOV) (Fig.4)

A 36-year-old female was referred to our hospital again after incomplete transarterial embolization of a cavernous DAVF. On admission, she suffered from slight exophthalmos and chemosis of her right eye. A cerebral angiogram demonstrated a residual arteriovenous shunt of the right CS supplied by the right meningohypophyseal trunk draining to the right SOV.

http://dx.doi.org/10.5772/56732

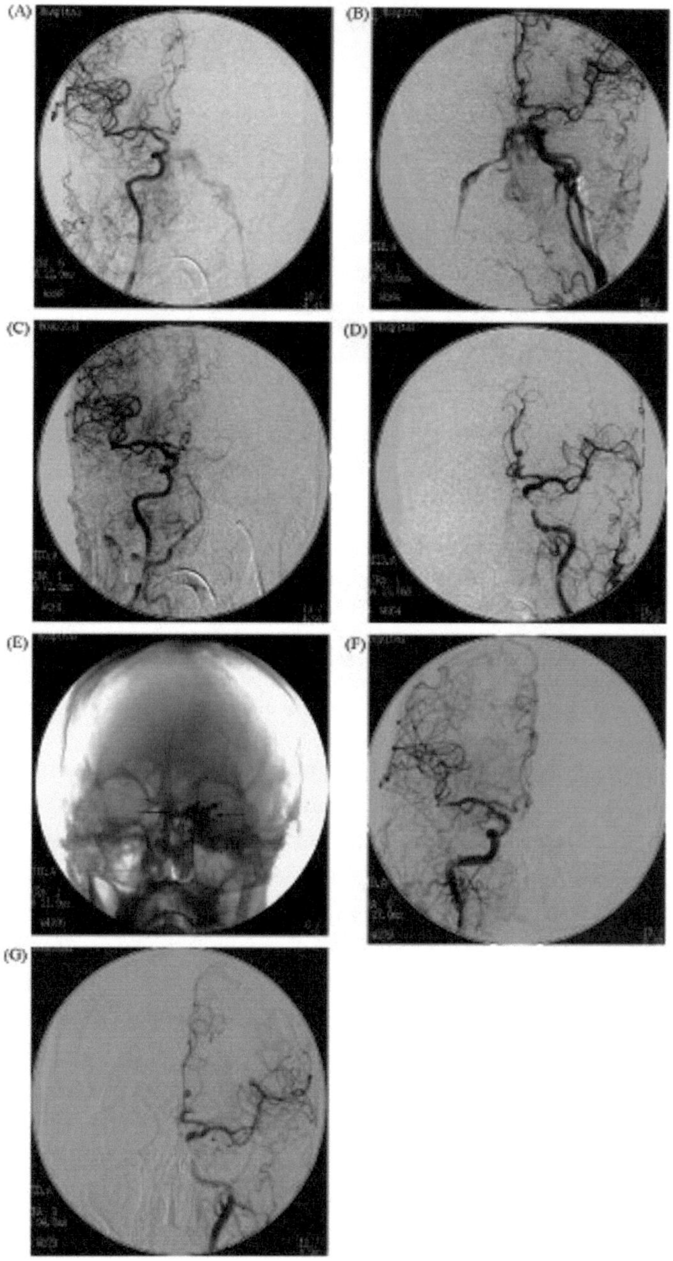

Figure 2. Right ICA angiogram, anteroposterior projection (A), left ICA angiogram, anteroposterior projection (B), show fed by both ICAs, mainly drained to left IPS and left SOV. Right ICA angiogram, anteroposterior projection (C) and left ECA angiogram, anteroposterior projedtion (D), after embolization showing the DAVF is completely occluded. (E) Skull X-ray film after embolization, anteroposterior projection, showing the Onyx cast (arrows). The follow-up angiographic study after 7 months, right CCA (F) and left CCA angiogram (G), demonstrated no recannalization of the fistula.

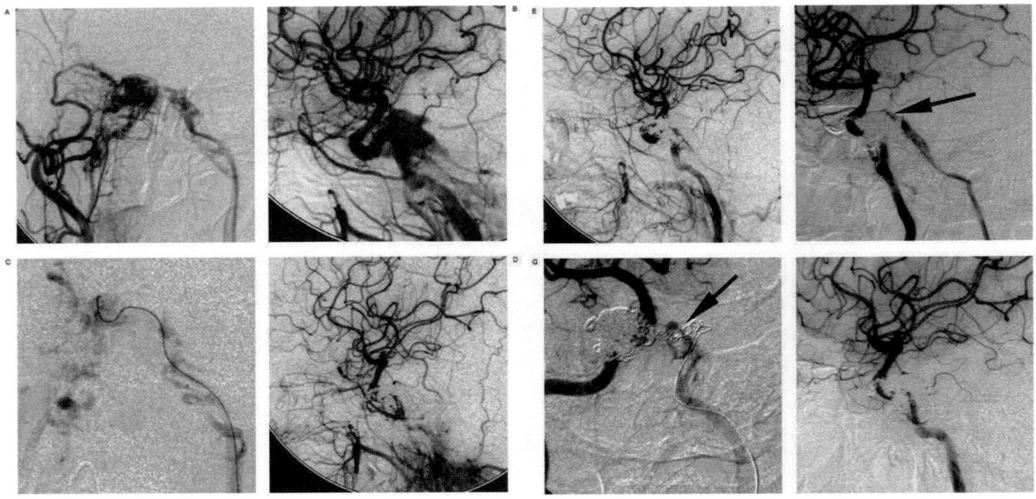

Figure 3. Right CCA angiogram, anteroposterior projection (A), left CCA angiogram, lateral projection (B), showing a CDAVF fed by both internal and external carotid arteries, mainly drained to the left IPS and the right SOV. Frontal superselective angiogram of the right CS (C), showing the microcatheter positioned close to the fistula site. After embolization, anterograms of the right common carotid artery (lateral view) (D) and left common carotid artery (lateral view) (E), demonstrating complete occlusion of the fistula. F, six months later, lateral angiogram of the right ICA, showing persistent filling of the residural fistula (arrow). G, occlusion of the intercavernous sinus (arrow), with several standard coils. H, angiogram of the right ICA (lateral view) after complete embolization of the right-side fistula.

The right facial vein and the right superficial temporal vein were demonstrated angiographically draining the fistula. Because the approach of superficial temporal vein was longer and tortuous, we decided to approach the right CS through the right facial vein. A 5-French guiding catheter (Envoy; Cordis Endovascular System) was advanced through the right internal jugular vein into the right common trunk of facial and retromandibular veins. A diagnostic catheter was placed in the right ICA via the left common femoral artery. A Marathon microcatheter was advanced through the guiding catheter and through the right facial vein into the right SOV. After traversing the SOV, we gain access to the right CS. Occlusion of the fistula was accomplished by filling the right CS with 1.5ml Onyx-34. In the meantime caution was exerted to avoid inadvertent embolization of the ICA during the slow injection of Onyx. Patency of the right ICA was checked frequently during the intermittent injection of the embolic material. There were no complications during the procedure. She was discharged 3 days after the procedure with symptoms improved.

3.5. Case report V:Cavernous DAVF (Direct puncture of SOV) (Fig.5)

A 43-year-old woman had a 2 month history of intracranial bruits, proptosis and chemosis of the right eye. Her vision was normal. An angiogram revealed a CS DAVF draining anteriorly into the enlarged right SOV. The fistula was fed by the meningeal branches of the right ECA and ICA, making it a Barrow type D DAVF. Because of progressive ocular symptoms and intracranial bruits, transvenous embolization was indicated. No IPS was opacified from either

http://dx.doi.org/10.5772/56732

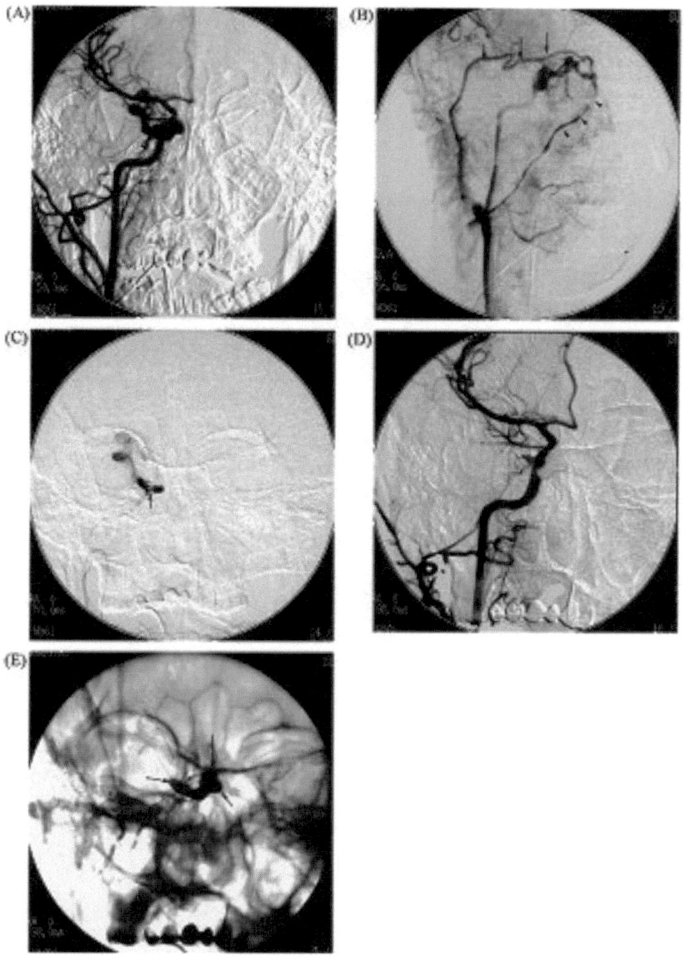

Figure 4. Right CCA angiogram, frontal projection (A), showing a DAVF involving the right CS fed by the left meningo-hypophyseal trunk and the right internal maxillary artery. Venous phase of the right CCA (B) demonstrated the venous drainage via the right IPS, the superficial temperal vein and the facial vein. Superselective angiography (C) showed the microcatheter in the right CS. Right CCA angiogram, frontal projection (D), showing the right CS completely packed. Skull X-ray film, frontal projection (E) showing the deposited Onyx in the right CS.

side, and cannulation of either IPS or the facial vein was not successful. Therefore, we recommended surgical exposure and direct cannulation of the right SOV, which was performed in the angiographic suite, as detailed above. A microcatheter was introduced through the trocar sheath, and several platinum coils were deployed into the CS to reduce the flow volume of the fistula. Then, Onyx was used to obliterate the CS until there was no filling of the CS. Final follow-up angiograms showed complete obliteration of the fistula. Postoperatively, her vision remained normal and the proptosis and chemosis improved within 5 days, and the patient's intracranial bruits also resolved. A 3 month follow-up angiogram showed durable complete occlusion of the CSDF. The eyelid incision healed well with excellent cosmesis.

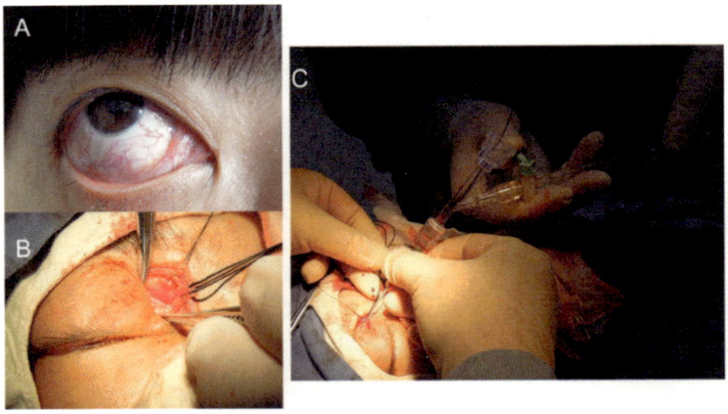

Figure 5. A) The patient presented with proptosis, chemosis and intracranial bruits caused by a cavernous sinus dural fistula. (B) A 2 cm subbrow incision was made in the upper medial eyelid crease on the affected side. A 10-15 mm segment of the SOV was isolated and controlled with 3-0 silk sutures and an intraoperative angiogram was performed to confirm the SOV. (C) An 18 size trocar was used to acupuncture the SOV, then moving the needle core, the trocar sheath was connected to a Y shaped valve. An Echelon-10 microcatheter was introduced through the tube.

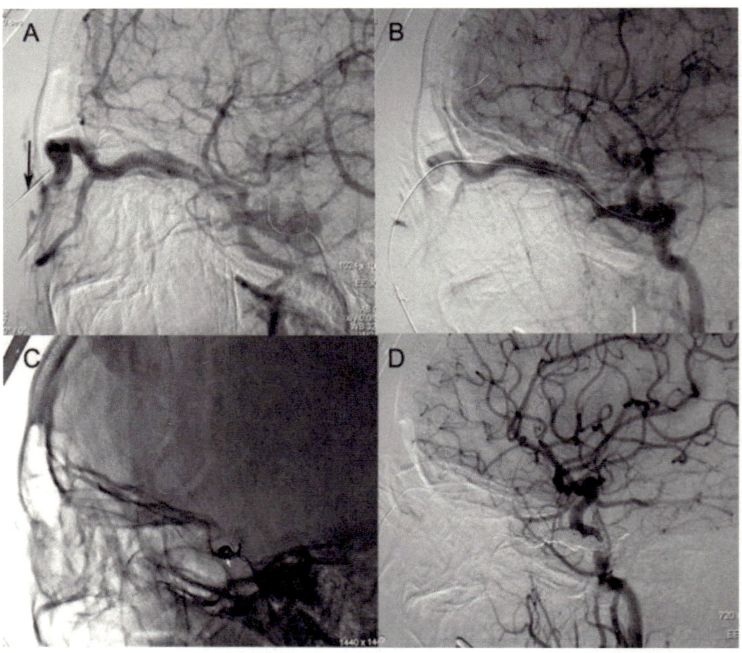

Figure 6. A) Later cerebral angiogram showing a CS dural fistula (Barrow type D) with anterior venous drainage in an enlarged right SOV. Note a metal landmark (arrow) was used to confirm the exposed SOV by transfemoral angiography. (B) The affected cavernous sinus was catheterized with an Echelon-10 microcatheter. Multiple coils (C) and Onyx (D) were deployed through the microcatheter to obliterate the cavernous sinus and proximal portion of the right SOV. The fistula was cured.

3.6. Case report VI:Transverse sigmoid sinus DAVF (Fig.7)

A 56-year-old man with headaches and pulsitile tinnitus demonstrated a left TSS Cognard Type IIa DAVF (Table1). An ophthalmological examination revealed bilateral papilledema. Cerebral angiography demonstrated multiple feeders arising from the left ECA and ICA and basal artery system with a parallel venous channel. One transarterial and one transvenous embolization of the TSS DAVF were performed. These procedures and occlusion of the ECA feeders significantly reduced the size of the fistula. After transvenous embolization of the left TSS, control angiography demonstrated obliteration of the parallel channel, with preservation of the patent parent sinus (Cognard Type I). During the subsequent months the patient's tinnitus was in stable condition and no further neurological symptoms were noted, ophthalmological examination was not available.

I Venous drainage into dural venous sinus with antegrade flow
IIa Venous drainage into dural venous sinus with retrograde flow
IIb Venous drainage into dural venous sinus with antegrade flow and CVR
IIa+b Venous drainage into dural venous sinus with retrograde flow and CVR
III Venous drainage directly into subarachnoid veins (CVR only)
IV Type III with venous ectasias of the draining subarachnoid veins

Table 1. Cognard classification of dural AVS (1995)

3.7. Case report VII:Tentorial DAVF (Fig.8)

A 70-year-old man presented with a headache of sudden onset and vomiting. Computed tomography demonstrated diffuse subarachnoid hemorrhage and a venous aneurysm at the right petrous apex. Selective right ECA and ICA angiography revealed a dural fistula supplied by branches of the right middle meningeal artery, ascending pharyngeal artery and tentorial branches of the right ICA. The fistula drained in the region of the right petrosal venous complex and thence into the basal vein to the straight sinus. There was a venous aneurysm appropriately 1 cm in diameter on the basal vein. We initially attempted ECA embolization. A microcatheter was placed in the posterior branch of the right middle meningeal artery and embolizing with 5-0 (1.0-1.5cm long) sutures. The ECA suppliers were occluded. But the fistula was still persistent and fed by the branches of the right asending pharyngeal artery and right ICA. We therefore decided on endovascular treatment using a transvenous approach. A microcatheter was placed in the right jugular vein was catheterized and a microcatheter was directed through the straight sinus into the basal vein. The venous varix was crossed with care and the tip of the microcatheter was placed at the site of the fistula in the petrosal venous complex. Using the venous catheter, five EDCs were then placed at the site of the fistula via the transvenous microcatheter. Angiography revealed complete occlusion of the fistula on both the ECA and ICA injections. The patient made an uneventful recovery. After 4 months, the follow-up angiograms of bilateral CCAs confirmed the complete obliteration and the patient demonstrated no symptoms.

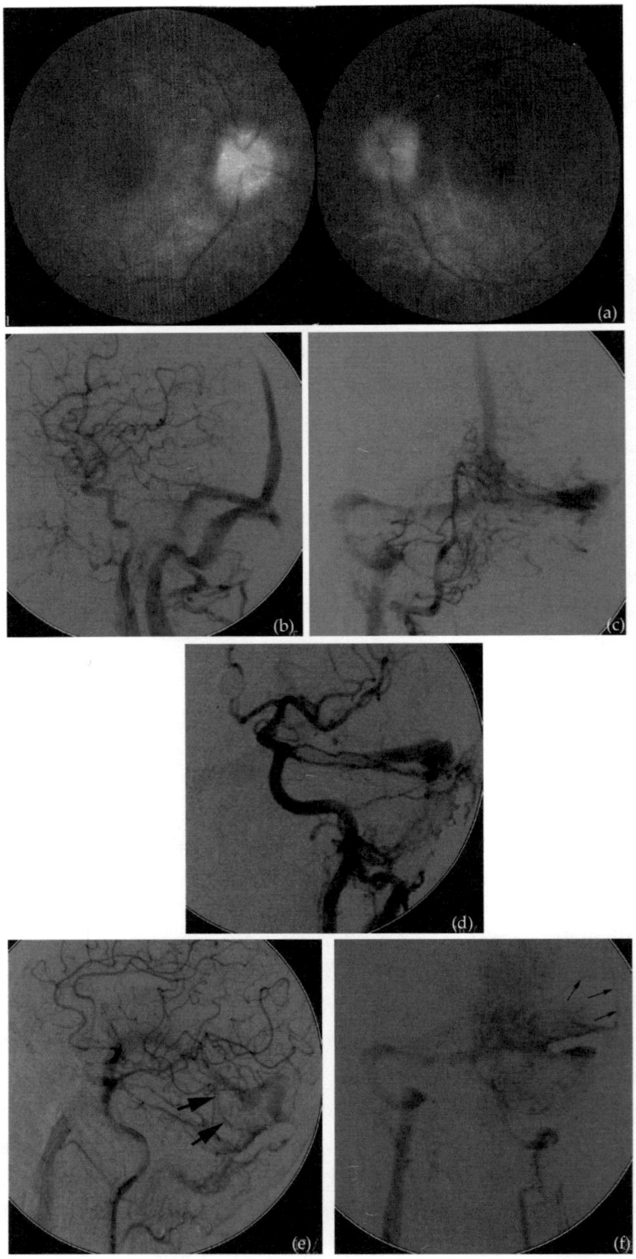

Figure 7. A, an ophthalmological examination revealed bilateral papilledema. B, ateriogram of the left CCA (arterial phase, lateral view), showing multiple feeders arising from the ICA and ECA. C, arteriogram of the right vertebral artery (arterial phase, frontal view), showing multiple feeders arising from the vertebral artery. D, the microcatheter was navigated into the left TSS via the right IJV-TSS. E-F, arteriograms (lateral view) of the left CCA (E) and left VA. The residual fistula was Cognard Type I with parallel venous channel was coiled and the parent sinus was patent, with preservation of the venous outflow (arrows) of the temporal lobe through the vein of Labbe.

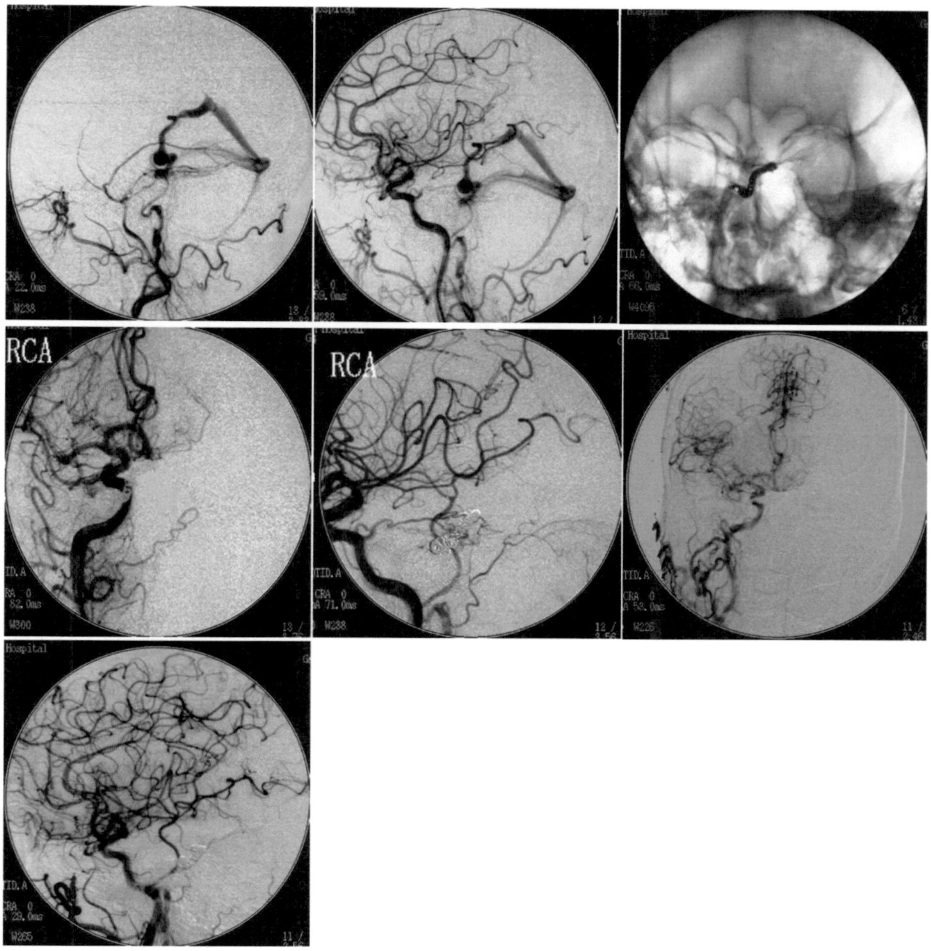

Figure 8. A, Lateral DSA of right ECA shows the fistula supplied by branches of the right middle meningeal artery and asending pharyngeal artery. B, Lateral DSA of the right CCA shows the meningohypophyseal trunk suppling the DAVF and the suppliers from the right meningeal artery were occluded. C, During procedure, the skull X-ray film shows the delivery of the detachable coils. Postprocedure angiograms of right CCA, frontal (D) and lateral (E), demonstrated complete obliteration of the fistula. Four-month after endovascular treatment, lateral DSAs of right CCA (F) and left CCA (G) show permanent occlusion of DAVF.

4. Discussion

Depending on their venous drainage patterns, intracranial DAVFs can cause headaches, dementia, chemosis, proptosis, bruit, and, rarely, infarction or hemorrhage. The data of our patients confirmed previous studies. [3, 6, 11, 37, 45, 51, 52] The clinical presentation is closely related to the degree of shunting, cerebral venous hypertension, and the pattern of venous drainage, with or without impaired cortical function. [1] Despite spontaneous remission, which occurs in 9.4 to 50% of cases, according to the literature, [20] treatment is indicated in cases with cortical drainage (Cognard Type IIb or greater), hemorrhage, progressive neurological deficits, or intractable headaches or tinnitus. Although cure rate of DAVFs of transarterial embolization has been promoted by Onyx, it is limited in smaller arteriovenous fistula DAVFs. [33] Transvenous embolization is still a good option for DAVFs with multiple feeding arteries, especially for transarterial embolization cannot be cured. [17-19] When transvenous catheterization is possible, transvenous embolization is associated with a high rate of permanent long-term occlusion. Occlusion can be achieved with placement of coils, via a transvenous route. Isobutyl-2-cyanoacrylate embolization, particles of polyvinyl alcohol or a detachable balloon have been used to pack the cavernous sinus before advancement of GDC.

5. Transvenous embolization of CS

There are different transvenous route to the CS, i.e., by way of the IPS, contralateral IPS, basilar plexus, or circular sinus, through the facial vein, angular vein, and SOV, or through the pterygoid plexus. [10, 12-14, 17, 23-28, 32, 50-54] To achieve complete occlusion, the cavernous sinus was tightly packed with GDC. This tight packing may have accounted for the intense nausea and vomiting. Transient VIth or IIIrd nerve palsy following coil embolization for cavernous DAVF are well-known events. [52] The complex nature of the fistula, the unexpected hardship in the placement of detachable coils, and our previous experience with Onyx in the treatment of DAVFs promoted us to use Onyx in the treatment of our patient. [11, 17, 18]

6. Transvenous embolization of DAVFs in other locations

For DAVFs in the ACF, we prefer transvenous procedure with softest EDC and free coils to fit the draining frontal veins and to minimize the risk of damage and rupture of the frontal veins, appreciating the risk of visual compromise from embolic occlusion of the central retinal artery. Although venous approach through the elongated, ectactic, and potentially fragile pial veins is considered difficult and risky, several cases of tentorial DAVF have been treated by transvenous embolization. [14, 19, 21]

If the affected TSS is isolated or exhibits prominent retrograde drainage to the cortical veins and is not a functional part of the venous circulation, then sinus occlusion via an endovascular. If there was anterograde flow in the vein of Labbe in a case of a lateral sinus fistula, the vein of Labbe should be spared after transvenous embolization of the TSS.

Kubo et al. [48] concluded, on the basis of their three cases and a review of the literature, that second fistulae can occur after complete embolization, with latency periods of more than one year and this finding was confirmed by Kiyosue et al. [9] For this reason, we occluded all main feeding arteries prior to obliteration of the affected sinus in our cases with DAVFs of tentorium and TSS to prevent development of cortical venous reflux and intracranial hemorrhage. In one patient with a TSS DAVF with a parallel venous channel of the transverse/sigmoid sinus was converted a Cognard Type IIa DAVF into a Cognard Type I DAVF with patent parent sinus.

7. Conclusion

Transvenous treatment of intracranial DAVFs can be a highly effective method if various transvenous approaches are attempted. Onyx is a promising embolic agent for the transvenous treatment of DAVFs, and its physical properties warrant further appraisal in larger series of patients. The advantages make this an attractive alternative to already described various platinum coils.

Author details

Xianli Lv, Youxiang Li and Chuhan Jiang*

*Address all correspondence to: lvxianli000@163.com

Beijing Neurosurgical Institute and Beijing Tiantan Hospital, Capital Medical University, Beijing, P R China

References

[1] Paula-Lucas C, Pereica-Caldas J-G-M, Prandini MN (2006)Do leptomeningeal venous drainage and dysplastic venous dilation predict hemorrhage in dural arteriovenous fistula? Surg Neurol 66:S3:2-S3:6

[2] Roy D, Raymond J (1997)The role of transvenous embolization in the treatment of intracranial dural arteriovenous fistulas. Neurosurgery 40 (6):1133-1144

[3] Urtasun F, Biondi A, Casaco A, Houdart E, Caputo N, Aymard A, Merland JJ (1996)Cerebral dural arteriovenous fistulas: percutaneous transvenous embolization. Radiology 199:209-217

[4] Cognard C, Gobin YP, Pierot L, Bailly AL, Houdart E, Casasco A, Chiras J, Merlland JJ (1995)Cerebral dural arteriovenous fistulas:clinical and angiographic correlation with a revised classification of venous drainage. Radiology 194:671-680

[5] Abrahams JM, Begley LJ, Flamm ES, Hurst RW, Sinson GP (2002)Alternative management considerations for ethmoidal dural arteriovenous fistula. Surgical Neurology 58 (6):410-417

[6] Benndorf G, Schmidt S, Sollman WP, Kroppenstedt SN (2003)Tentorial dural arteriovenous fistula presenting with various visual symptoms related to anterior and posterior visual pathway dysfunction: case report. Neurosurgery 53:222-227

[7] Halbach VV, Higashida RT, Hieshima GR, Wilson CB, Barnwell SL, Dowd CF (1990)Dural arteriovenous fistulas supplied by ethmoidal arteries. Neurosurgery 26:816-823

[8] Iwamuro Y, Nakahara I, Higashi T, Iwaasa M, Watanabe Y, Hirata E, Tsunetoshi K, Taha M (2006)Tentorial dural arteriovenous fistula presenting symptoms due to mass effect on the dilated draining vein: case report. Surg Neurol 65:511-515

[9] Kim MS, Han DH, Han MH, Oh C-W (2003)Posterior fossa hemorrhage caused by dural arteriovenous fistula: case reports. Surg Neurol 59:512-517

[10] Leonard F, Jeffrey B, Nicholas JV (2003)Cavernous sinus fistulas: carotid cavernous fistulas and dural arteriovenous malformations. Current Neurology & Neuroscience Reports 3:415-420

[11] Lv X, Li Y, Wu Z (2008)Endovascular treatment of the anterior cranial fossa dural arteriovenous fistulas. Neuroradiology 50:433-437

[12] Arat A, Cekirge S, Saatci I, Ozgen B (2004)Transvenous injection of Onyx for casting of the cavernous sinus for the treatment of a carotid-cavernous fistula. Neuroradiology 46:1012-1015

[13] Benndorf G, Bender A, Lehmann R, Lanksch W (2000)Transvenous occlusion of dural cavernous sinus fistulas through the thrombosed inferior petrosal sinus: report of four cases and review of the literature. Surg Neurol 54:42-54

[14] Deasy NP, Gholkar AR, Cox TCS, Jeffree MA (1999)Tentorial dural arteriovenous fistulas: endovascular treatment with transvenous coil embolization. Neuroradiology 41:308-312

[15] Defreyne L, Vanlangenhove P, Vandekerckhove T, Deschrijver I, Sieben G, Klaes R, Kunnen M (2000)Transvenous embolization of a dural arteriovenous fistula of the anterior cranial fossa:preliminary results. AJNR Am J Neuroradiol 21:761-765

[16] Jahan R, Gobin YP, Glenn B, Duckwiler GR, Vinuela F (1998)Transvenous embolization of a dural arteriovenous fistula of the cavernous sinus through the contralateral pterygoid plexus. Neuroradiology 40:189-193.

[17] Jiang C, Lv X, Li Y, Liu A, Lv M, Jiang P, Wu Z (2007)Transvenous Embolization of Cavernous Sinus Dural Arteriovenous Fistula with Onyx-18 and Plentinum coils: Technical Note. NRJ-Neuroradiol J. 20:47-52

[18] Jiang C, Lv X, Li Y, Liu A, Wu Z (2007)Transvenous embolization with Onyx for dural arteriovenous fistula of cavernous sinus: a report of two case reports. NRJ-Neuroradiol J. 20:718-725

[19] Jiang C, Lv X, Li Y, Wu Z (2007)Transarterial and transvenous embolization for tentorial dural arteriovenous fistula: case report. NRJ-Neuroradiol J 20:726-729

[20] Kai Y, Hamada J, Morioka M, Yano S, Kuratsu J (2007)Treatment of cavernous sinus dural arteriovenous fistulas by external manual carotid compression. Neurosurgery 60:253-258

[21] Kajita Y, Miyachi S, Wakabayashi T, Inao S, Yoshida J (1999)A dural arteriovenous fistula of the tentorium successfully treated by intravascular embolization. Surg Neurol 52:294-298

[22] Kallmes DF, Jensen ME, Kassell NF, Dion JE (1997)Percutaneous transvenous coil embolization of a Djindjian type 4 tentorial dural arteriovenous malformation. AJNR Am J Neuroradiol 18:673-676.

[23] Kazekawa K, Iko M, Sakamoto S, Aikawa H, Tsutsumi M, Kodama T, Go Y, Tanaka A (2003)Dural AVFs of the cavernous sinus: transvenous embolization using a direct superficial temporal vein approach. Radiation Medicine 21:138-141

[24] Kuwayama N, Endo S, Kitabayashi M, Nishijima M, Takaku A (1998)Surgical transvenous embolization of a cortically draining carotid cavernous fistula via a vein of the sylvian fissure. AJNR Am J Neuroradiol 19 (7):1329-1332.

[25] Lefkowitz M, Giannotta SL, Hieshima G, Higashida R, Halbach V, Dowd C, Teitelbaum GP (1998)Embolization of neurosurgical lesions involving the ophthalmic artery. Neurosurgery 43:1298-1303

[26] Liu HM, Huang YC, Wang YH, Tu YK (2000)Transarterial embolization of complex cavernous sinus dural arteriovenous fistulas with low-concentration cyanoacrylate. Neuroradiology 42:766-770.

[27] Nakamura M, Tamaki N, Kawaguchi T, Fujita S (1998)Selective transvenous embolization of dural carotid-cavernous sinus fistulas with preservation of sylvian venous outflow. Report of three cases. J. Neurosurg 89:825-829

[28] Oishi H, Arai H, Sato K, Iizuka Y (1999)Complications associated with transvenous embolization of cavernous dural arteriovenous fistula. Acta Neurochir 141:1265-1271

[29] Satomci J, Satoh K, Matsubara S, Nakajima N, Nagahiro S (2005)Angiographic changes in venous drainage of cavernous sinus dural arteriovenous fistulas after palliative transarterial embolization or observational management: a proposed stage classification. Neurosurgery 56:494-502.

[30] Siekmann R, Weber W, Kis B, Kuhne D (2005)Transvenous treatment of a dural arteriovenous fistula of the transverse sinus by embolization with platinum coils and Onyx HD 500+. Inter Neuroradiol 11:281-286

[31] So-Hyang I, Chang WO, Dae HH (2004)Surgical management of an unruptured dural arteriovenous fistula of the anterior cranial fossa: natural history for 7 year. Surg Neurol 62:72-75.

[32] Suzuki S, Lee DW, Jahan R, Duckwiler GR, Vinuela F (2006)Transvenous treatment of spontaneous dural carotid-cavernous fistulas using a combination of detachable coils and Onyx. AJNR Am J Neuroradiol 27:1346-1349

[33] Toulgoat F, Mounayer C, Tulio Salles Rezende M, Piotin M, Spelle L, Lazzarotti G, Desal H, Moret J (2006)Transarterial embolization of intracranial dural arteriovenous malformations with ethylene vinyl alcohol copolymer (Onyx-18). J Neuroradiol 33:105-114

[34] Troffkin NA, Graham CB, Berkman T, Wakhloo AK (2003)Combined transvenous and transarterial embolization of a tentorial-incisural dural arteriovenous malformation followed by primary stent placement in the associated stenotic straight sinus. Case report. J. Neurosurg 99 (3):579-583.

[35] Tu YK, Liu HM, Hu SC (1997)Direct surgery of carotid cavernous fistulas and dural arteriovenous malformations of the cavernous sinus. Neurosurgery 41 (4):798-806.

[36] Watanabe T, Matsumaru Y, Sonobe M, Asahi T, Onitsuka K, Sugita K, Takahashi S, Nose T (2000)Multiple dural arteriovenous fistulas involving the cavernous and sphenoparietal sinuses. Neuroradiology 42:771-774.

[37] Deshmukh VR, Maughan PH, Spetzler RF (2006)Resolution of hemifacial spasm after surgical obliteration of a tentorial arteriovenous fistula: case report. Neurosurgery 58 (1):E202

[38] Deshmukh VR, Maughan PH, Spetzler RF (2006)Resolution of hemifacial spasm after surgical obliteration of a tentorial arteriovenous fistula: case report. Neurosurgery 58 (1):E202

[39] Fujita A, Tamaki N, Nakamura M, Yosuo K, Morikawa M (2001)A tentorial dural arteriovenous fistula successfully treated with interruption of leptomeningeal venous drainage using microvascular Doppler sonography: case report. Surg Neurol 56:56-61.

[40] Jesus OD, Rosado JE (1999)Tentorial dural arteriovenous fistula obliteration using the petrosal approach. Surg Neurol 51:164-167.

[41] Komotar RJ (2007)Clinicoradiological review: bilateral ethmoidal artery dural arteriovenous fistulas. Neurosurgery 60 (1):131-136

[42] Mayfrank L, Reul J, Huffmann B, BertalanHy H, Spetzger U, Gilsbach JM (1996)Microsurgical interhemispheric approach to dural arteriovenous fistulas of the floor of the anterior cranial fossa. Minimally Invasive Neurosurgery 39 (3):74-77.

[43] White DV, Sincoff EH, Abdulrauf SI (2005)Anterior ethmoidal artery: mirosurgical anatomy and ethmoidal considerations. Neurosurgery 56 (4)ONS (2):406-410.

[44] Masahiro S, Hiroki K, Masao T, Takaaki K (2000)Stereotactic radiosurgery for tentorial dural arteriovenous fistulas draining into the vein of Galen: reports of two cases. Neurosurgery 46 (3):730

[45] Matsushige T, Nakaoka M, Ohta K, Yahara K, Okamotor H, Kurisu K (2006)Tentorial dural arteriovenous malformation manifesting as trigeminal neuralgia treated by stereotactic radiosurgery: a case report. Surg Neurol 66:519-523

[46] Pannu Y, Shownkeen H, Nockels RP, Origitano TC (2004)Obliteration of a tentorial dural arteriovenous fistula causing spinal cord myelopathy using the cranio-orbital zygomatic approach. Surg Neurol 62:463-467.

[47] Patrik RT, Harry JC, Akihiko K, Micheal CC, Jacques D, Daniel LB (2003)Evolution of the management of tentorial dural arteriovenous malformations. Neurosurgery 52 (4):750-762.

[48] Kong DS, Kwon KH, Kim JS, Hong SC, Jeon P (2007)Combined surgical approach with intraoperative endovascular embolization for inaccessible dural arteriovenous fistulas. Surg Neurol 68:72-78

[49] Krisht AF, Burson T (1999)Combined pretemporal and endovascular approach to the cavernous sinus for the treatment of carotid-cavernous dural fistulas: technical case report. Neurosurgery 44 (2):415-418.

[50] Quinones D, Duckwiler G, Gobin PY, Goldberg RA, Vinuela F (1997)Embolization of dural cavernous fistulas via superior ophthalmic vein approach. AJNR Am J Neuroradiol 18:921-928

[51] Kim DJ, Kim DI, Suh SH, Kim J, Lee SK, Kim EY, Chung TS (2006)Results of transvenous embolization of cavernous dural arteriovenous fistula: A single-center experience with emphasis on complications and management. AJNR Am J Neuroradiol 27 (10):2078-2082

[52] Aihara N, Mase M, Yamada K, Barno T, Watanake K, Kamiya K, Takagi T (1999)Deterioration of ocular motor dysfunction after transvenous embolization of dural arteriovenous fistula involving the cavernous sinus. Acta Neurochir 141:707-710.

[53] Benndorf G, Bender A, Campi A, Menneking H, Lanksch WR (2001)Treatment of a cavernous sinus dural arteriovenous fistula by deep orbital puncture of the superior ophthalmic vein. Neuroradiology 43:499-502

[54] Goldberg RA, Goldey SH, Duckwiler G, Vineula F (1997)Management of cavernous sinus-dural fistulas. Indications and techniques for primary embolization via the superior ophthalmic vein. Arch Ophthamol 115:823-824

Section 2

Spinal Arteriovenous Fistula

Chapter 3

Spinal Arteriovenous Lesions

Benjamin Brown, Chiazo Amene, Shihao Zhang,
Sudheer Ambekar, Hugo Cuellar and
Bharat Guthikonda

Additional information is available at the end of the chapter

http://dx.doi.org/10.5772/56731

1. Introduction

Spinal arteriovenous lesions represent a heterogeneous set of pathologic entities. As our general understanding of these lesions has evolved, so have the classification systems clinicians use to describe them. Historically, the most common classification of arteriovenous fistulas (AVF) has been the Type I-IV classification. More recently these lesions have been described from an anatomical and physiologic perspective.

This text will use the most recent categorizations by Spetzler, et al in 2002 [15]. Table 1 provides an overview of the spinal arteriovenous lesions discussed in this chapter and can be used as a quick reference for comparison.

2. Extradural arteriovenous fistulae

2.1. Anatomy/etiology/classification

The extradural arteriovenous fistulae represent an abnormal connection between an epidural artery and the epidural venous plexus, otherwise known as Batson's plexus [2]. This connection produces engorgement of the epidural plexus and subsequent mass effect upon the thecal sac and spinal cord within [10]. Venous drainage can be confined to the epidural space or may reflux into the perimedullary veins [28]. These fistulae occur more commonly in the thoracic and lumbar spine than the cervical spine. The cause of these lesions is unknown, though both post-surgical and post-traumatic lesions have been documented [18, 26-27]. These have been referred to as epidural fistulas in previous classification schemes and are not included in the

	Extradural	Dorsal Intradural	Ventral Intradural	Intramedullary	Extradural-Intradural	Conus Medullaris
Pathophysiology	Compression, venous congestion, vascular steal	Venous congestion	Compression, hemorrhage, vascular steal	Compression, vascular steal, hemorrhage	Compression, vascular steal, hemorrhage	Compression, vascular steal, hemorrhage
Presentation	Myelopathy	Myelopathy	Myelopathy	Pain, acute myelopathy	Pain, myelopathy	Myelopathy, radiculopathy
Flow	High	Low	High	High	High	Variable
Nidus	Extradural artery and vein	Radicular artery to medullary vein at root sleeve	Pial surface	Spinal cord parenchyma	Diffuse: Extradural, intradural, parenchymal, muscle, bone	Multiple feeders from anterior and posterior spinal arteries
Alternate Nomenclature	Epidural fistulas	Type IA, Spinal dural AVF, Dural AVF	Type IV, anterior intradural AVF, or Perimedullary AVF	Type II, Classic AVM, or Glomus	Type III, Metameric, or Juvenile	None

Table 1. Overview of Spinal Arteriovenous Lesions

Type I-IV dural AVF classification. Rangel-Castilla et al proposed subdividing extradural arteriovenous fistulae into three types: A, B1, and B2. Type A fistulae have at least one intradural draining vein, while types B1 and B2 have purely extradural drainage. Type B1 has mass effect on the thecal sac, while in type B2 there is no mass effect by the distended epidural veins [28].

2.2. Clinical manifestation

Due to their rarity, it is difficult to provide epidemiological data on extradural arteriovenous fistulae. Case reports suggest their average age of presentation to be in the seventh decade of life [27-28]. Clinically, they result in a progressive myelopathy [15]. This is thought to be secondary to direct mass effect from engorged veins as well as intramedullary venous hypertension secondary to poor outflow [2]. The constellation of symptoms varies based on the location of lesion. Patients may experience a compressive radiculopathy or myelopathy. Venous hypertension may also lead to progressive myelopathy in a manner similar to dural AVF. Vascular steal is thought to play less of a role because these shunts do not involve afferents with associated arterial supply to the spinal cord [23].

2.3. Imaging

MRI examination reveals a picture identical to spinal dural AVF. There will be swelling in the parenchyma of the cord identified by T2 hyperintensity within the cord. Serpentine structures around the surface of the cord may be noted as T2 "flow-voids." Additionally there may be dural enhancement on T1 weighted imaging with contrast. Formal angiography remains the "gold standard" and will best delineate the anatomy of each individual extradural AVF.

2.4. Treatment

These lesions rarely require open surgery and are treated very effectively by endovascular procedures [15]. Most commonly the use of liquid embolic such as Onyx is used to arrest flow within the fistula. Rarely open microsurgery can be used when vascular access to a given lesion is not possible. Partial obliteration of these lesions may allow for the remaining AVF to recruit new blood vessels and recur, thus treatment aims to completely obliterate the lesion.

2.5. Outcomes

Due to the rarity of these lesions, reliable outcome data is not available. However, treatment usually halts and often reverses progression of symptoms.

3. Intradural AVFs

These can be divided into two types: Dorsal intradural AVFs and Ventral intradural AVFs.

4. Dorsal intradural AVFs

4.1. Anatomy/epidemiology

Dorsal intradural AVFs correspond to the classic 'Type I' lesions in the original nomenclature. They are the most common type of spinal AVF, making up about 70% of all spinal AV malformations [9]. There is a male predominance, approximately 5:1, and it is usually diagnosed in the 5th to 6th decades of life [5]. They are most commonly found in the thoracic and thoracolumbar regions (greater than 80%) [5, 9, 33], with approximately 2% in the cervical spine and 4% in the sacral region [5].

Dorsal intradural AVFs are formed by a pathologic connection between one or more radiculomeningeal arteries and the venous outflow. The radiculomeningeal artery supplies the corresponding nerve root and meninges but not necessarily the spinal cord parenchyma. The shunt is located intradurally at the level of the dural sleeve surrounding the nerve root and drains into the venous system [2]. They characteristically have slow flow [15] and may be grouped into 2 subtypes. Subtype A involves a single feeding artery while Subtype B involves multiple feeders that converge into a single fistula, still on the intradural side of the nerve root. Venous outflow obstruction appears to be a hallmark of this type of lesion and may contribute to the formation of the shunt. This type of AVF is acquired and is theorized to result from traumatic injury, infection, or prior surgery; although often, the causative agent is never identified.

4.2. Pathophysiology

The pathology seen in spinal AVF was first described in 1926 by Foix and Alajouanine [30]. They described a progressive subacute necrotizing myelopathy, now known as Foix-Alajouanine syndrome, and found evidence of vascular obstruction, spinal cord necrosis and tortuous and dilated vasculature on the surface of the spinal cord. The actual etiology of the noted pathology was not cemented until Aminoff and Logue proposed that spinal cord ischemia secondary to venous congestion or hypertension was the underlying cause. The venous hypertension results in arterialization of the coronal venous plexus [15] which in turn leads to a decreased pressure gradient between the artery and vein and, therefore, decreases drainage of the spinal cord. This results in progressive venous congestion and edema of the spinal cord parenchyma with progressive symptoms.

4.3. Clinical manifestation

Aminoff et al. also characterized the clinical presentation of their patients with spinal AVF. They noted a gradual progression of symptoms; additionally, they noted that in approximately 50% of cases, spinal AVF led to severe disability [32]. Early symptoms of dorsal intradural AVF are often non-specific which may lead to delay in diagnosis. The end result is a progressive myelopathy. Lower extremity weakness is the most common initial presenting symptom, seen in about 50% of cases [24], although patients often reported milder symptoms months to years prior to presentation. Other symptoms seen at presentation, in order of descending frequency, include gait disturbance, paresthesias, back pain and bladder or sexual dysfunction [24]. This type of SDAVF rarely presents with hemorrhage. Patients are often graded clinically based on the Aminoff-Logue Scale (ALS) (Table 2)

	Score
Gait	
Some leg weakness, but able to walk unaided	1
Restricted exercise tolerance	2
Requires a cane to walk	3
Requires 2 canes or crutches to walk	4
Requires a wheelchair, unable to stand	5
Micturation	
Normal	0
Hesitancy, urgency, frequency, altered sensation, but continent	1
Occasional urinary incontinence or retention	2
Total incontinence or persistent retention	3
Bowel	
Mild constipation	1
Occasional incontinence or persistent constipation	2
Persistent incontinence	3

Table 2. Aminoff-Logue Scale

http://dx.doi.org/10.5772/56731

4.4. Imaging

4.4.1. MRI

MRI is the initial image modality used in the evaluation of suspected dorsal intradural AVFs. MRI often reveals increased signal intensity at the center of the cord on T2-weighted images which corresponds to cord edema and which may span several levels. Dorsal intradural flow voids may be present and are more evident on T2-weighted images or contrast-enhanced T1-weighted images. With the advancement in MRI technology, MRA can more reliably identify the location of the fistula though spinal angiography remains the gold standard [8, 25]. (Figure 1)

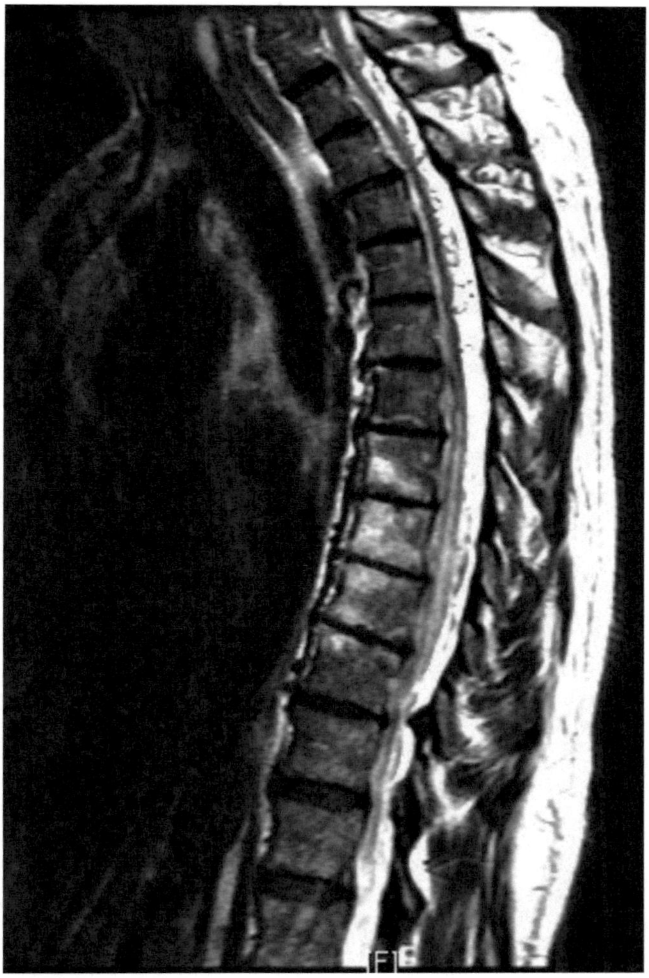

Figure 1. T2 Sagittal MRI showing tortuous vasculature on the dorsal aspect of the spinal cord and signal change within the cord representing edema.

4.4.2. Selective Spinal Angiography (SSA)

Even with the advances in MR imaging and angiography, catheter angiography remains the gold standard for diagnosis of dorsal intradural AVFs. It also provides an opportunity for possible endovascular treatment (discussed below). SSA reveals tortuous dilated vessels that may span many levels and also the characteristic slow-flow pattern produced by the feeding dorsal radiculomeningeal artery (Figure 2).

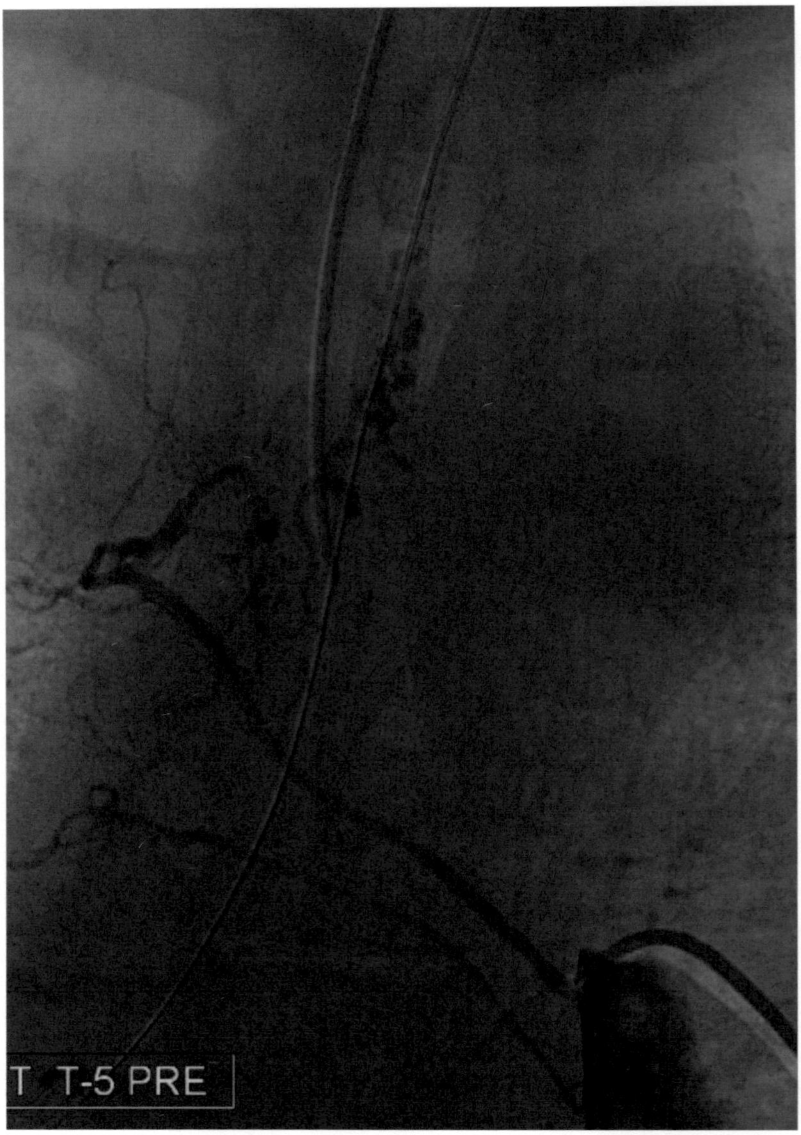

Figure 2. Spinal angiogram showing a dorsal intradural SDAVF filling from the right at T5

While SSA is still considered superior to other modes for diagnosis, it is not without potential complications. It often requires selective catheterization of many spinal feeders to determine the main feeding artery which results in lengthy procedures with extensive exposure to ionizing radiation and potential nephrotoxic levels of contrast agent [8]. Also due to the length of the procedures, it is often done with general anesthesia which presents its own complications. There have also been reports of neurologic injury caused by catheterization of spinal arteries.

4.5. Treatment

Secondary to the progressive nature of this disease, definitive and prompt treatment is required to halt the process.

4.5.1. Microsurgery

Historically, intradural dorsal AVFs were thought to be posterior angiomas and surgical treatment involved the stripping of dorsal perimedullary veins. This often resulted in worsening of neurologic function. It was discovered that instead, treating the intradural arterialized vein at the nerve root was the appropriate course of action. Therefore, surgery involves performing a hemilaminectomy, opening the dura, and following the dorsal radiculomeningeal artery as it heads towards the dorsal nerve root and ligating the artery-vein connection by coagulation or clipping. Surgery has been shown to be associated with very low morbidity (2%), with complete occlusion achieved in >98% of cases [17].

4.5.2. Endovascular

The recent advances in endovascular techniques have provided an alternative to surgical treatment of SDAVFs. It is less invasive, and may be performed at the same time as the diagnostic angiogram. Early endovascular endeavors utilized polyvinyl alcohol particulates to achieve obliteration of the fistula. However, this was complicated by high recanalization rates [19]. More recently, endovascular surgeons utilize liquid embolics like N-butylcyanoacrylate (NBCA) and Onyx. In some cases, embolization has been used as an adjunct to surgical resection. Embolization is contraindicated in cases where a spinal cord artery (radiculomedullary artery) arises from the same pedicle as the feeder. Attempts with endovascular treatment in these cases may result in either inadequate embolization or spinal cord ischemia if the medullary artery is occluded [5-6]. Embolization, even with liquid embolics, is still associated with high recurrence rates—up to 54% in the literature [17].

4.6. Outcomes

Prognosis after treatment directly correlates with duration and severity of pre-operative symptoms (6, 8, 31). Otherwise, there has been an inconsistency in the literature regarding prognosis after treatment. Clinical improvement of the motor function ranges from 25% to 100% [4, 31].

5. Ventral intradural AVFs

5.1. Anatomy/epidemiology:

These lesions correspond to 'Type IV' lesions in the classic categorization. In the literature, they are also referred to as perimedullary AVFs or fistulous arteriovenous malformations (AVMs). They are extremely rare, with only a few cases reported in the literature [14]. They occur in a younger population, with mean age in the 20's and 30's and no sex predilection [13-14]. They are also more prevalent at the conus medullaris and cauda equina [14].

Ventral intradural AVFs originate from the anterior spinal artery [14, 15]. The fistulous connection lies completely outside the cord parenchyma and pia matter in the subarachnoid space ventral to the cord at the midline. Blood flow through these AVFs is rapid and they may have flow-related aneurysms and venous hypertension [15]. In contrast to the dorsal types, ventral intradural AVFs may present as congenital lesions, but there is evidence supporting an acquired etiology to these lesions. They can be further subdivided into 3 distinct types based on feeding vessel size, shunt volume and drainage pattern [11, 15].

Type A – Small with a single feeder and low shunt volume. The feeding artery and draining vein are not significantly dilated. Hemodynamic features are similar to dorsal intradural AVFs.

Type B – These are of an intermediate size with a major feeder from anterior spinal artery as well as smaller feeders at the level of the fistula.

Type C – These are giant lesions with multi-pediculated and massively dilated venous channels and large shunt volumes. Hemodynamic features are similar to intramedullary AVMs.

5.2. Pathophysiology

Ventral intradural AVFs were first described by Djindjian in 1977 [12] and later classified as Type IV by Heros in 1986 [3]. They originate from the anterior spinal artery, with a direct fistulous connection to the engorged venous drainage system. There are no capillaries between the artery and the venous network. The pathology is similar to dorsal intradural AVFs with venous hypertension a common finding. However, the cause of the venous hypertension appears to be me more from vascular steal and mechanical compression [15] than from slow flow and venous congestion. Secondary to the higher flow rate through these AVFs, hemorrhage is more common and occurs in about 20-40% of cases [13-14].

5.3. Clinical manifestation

As opposed to the dorsal AVFs, symptoms are thought to be produced by vascular steal and mechanical compression from engorged veins or by subarachnoid or intraparenchymal hemorrhage. Symptoms are usually progressive in nature, with myelopathy the most common finding. Cases in which a patient may have an acute presentation or an acute exacerbation of baseline symptoms are usually a result of hemorrhage.

http://dx.doi.org/10.5772/56731

5.4. Imaging

5.4.1. MRI

MR Imaging is often the initial image modality used to diagnose ventral intradural AVFs. Like their dorsal counterparts, T2 prolongation in the parenchyma may be noted with flow voids on the ventral aspect of the cord or thecal sac. However, it is difficult to determine the type of AVF or differentiate between the subtypes of ventral AVFs and spinal angiography remains the standard for diagnosis. (Figure 3)

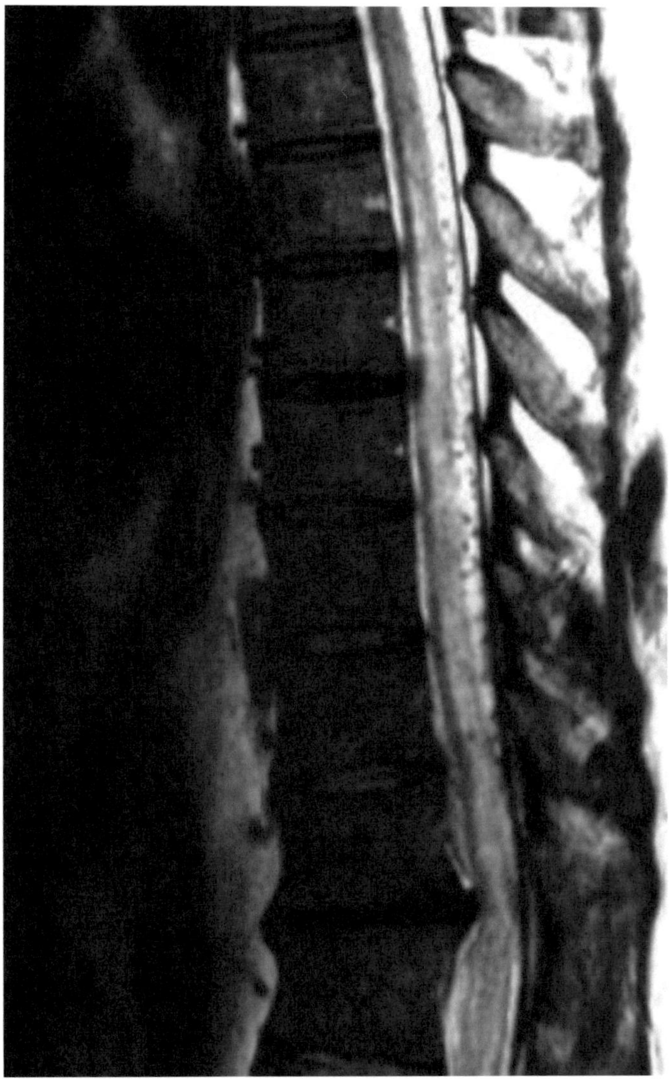

Figure 3. T2 Sagittal MRI showing hyperintensity within the spinal cord indicating edema

5.4.2. SSA

Catheterization of the anterior spinal artery cements the diagnosis of ventral intradural AVFs. (Figure 4)

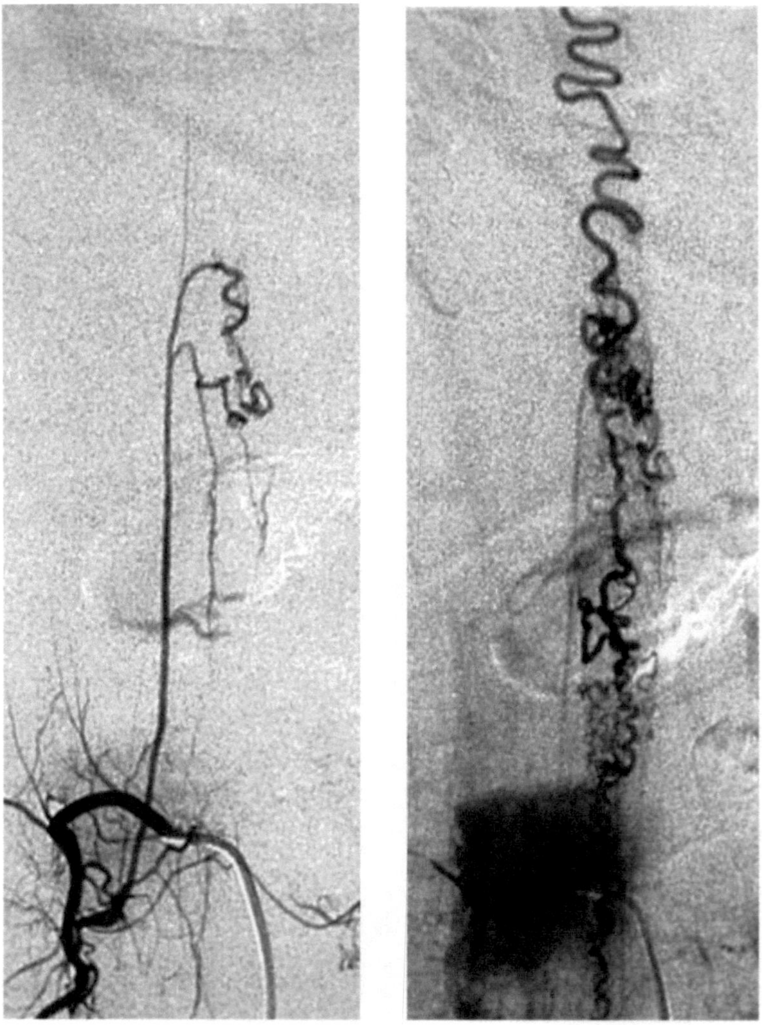

Figure 4. Spinal angiography showing an AVF fed by an anterior spinal artery at the thoracic level. Delayed images show the perispinal venous drainage of the fistula.

5.5. Treatment

Treatment modality depends on the subtype of the ventral intradural AVFs. Types A and B are often treated surgically, while Type C lesions are almost always treated via endovascular embolization [13-15].

5.5.1. Microsurgery

Surgery is the treatment of choice for Types A and B ventral intradural AVFs. This is feasible when they are located at the conus or cauda equina but may prove difficult in higher lesions and necessitate an anterior or anterolateral approach for treatment [14]. The target for surgery is the fistulous connection. Care must be taken to preserve the patency of the anterior spinal artery [2].

5.5.2. Endovascular

Endovascular embolization is often of limited use in these lesions due to the involvement of the anterior spinal artery, which is difficult to catheterize and navigate. For Type C lesions, however, endovascular treatment via embolization or detachable balloon occlusion appears to be the only safe course of action secondary to the large size of the lesion and easy catheterization of the severely dilated anterior spinal artery [2, 13-14].

5.6. Outcomes

Treatment usually results in stabilization of symptoms. Secondary to the paucity of these cases in the literature, definitive prognostic figures are not available.

6. Extradural-intradural arteriovenous malformations

Extradural-Intradural Arteriovenous Malformation is rare and very complex. It has been called type III, metameric, or juvenile AVM. It contains an intramedullary nidus which may take up the entire spinal canal at the occupied level. It could involve bony, extradural, intradural, and intramedullary tissue. This is a high-flow system with multiple feeding and draining vessels. The cause of this malformation is thought to be a problem with embryogenesis [2, 15, 37].

6.1. Clinical manifestations

Adolescents and young adults are the most affected by this type of AVM. Patients usually present with pain or progressive myelopathic symptoms from spinal cord compression, venous hypertension, or vascular steal. Intramedullary or subarachnoid hemorrhage could also lead to meningismus or acute pain [15, 37]. While only 35% of patients present with hemorrhage, over 50% have multiple hemorrhage at the time of diagnosis.

6.2. Imaging

MRI is the modality of choice when determining the location of the AVM. Flow voids can be seen on T1 weighted imaging. On T2 weighted imaging, hyperintensity and cord expansion are noted, which may be associated with venous hypertension. Appearance of subarachnoid or intraparenchymal bleeding on MRI varies depending on whether it is acute or chronic blood. In extradural-intradural AVM, the extension of the vessels into the paraspinal tissue can be found on MRI [2, 15, 37].

6.3. Treatment

The goal for treating extradural-intradural AVM is no different than any other type of AVM —obliteration of the nidus without causing damage to the spinal cord. However, treatment is very difficult and involves a multidisciplinary approach. A common strategy is to embolize the multiple feeding arteries followed by resecting the nidus if possible. Complete resection without neurological deficits is extremely difficult [15, 20, 37].

6.4. Outcome

Many cases of extradural-intradural AVM are inoperable. There are only a few case reports that relate successful resection of nidus with pre-operative embolization. No long term outcome data is available for this disorder [20].

7. Intramedullary AVM's

7.1. Anatomy and etiology

A spinal intramedullary AVM is formed by multiple abnormal vessels constituting a nidus with a feeding artery and a draining vein. These lesions were classified as type II (glomus) AVMs in the earlier classification by Anson and Spetzler [11] and as intramedullary AVMs in a later classification [15]. The nidus may be entirely intramedullary in location, intra and extramedullary or may be located in the region of conus medullaris. The intramedullary AVMs resemble the intracranial AVMs closely, in that they are located within the parenchyma and have distinct multiple feeding arteries from either the anterior or posterior spinal arteries and draining veins. These lesions are most often located in the cervico-thoracic area. Another distinct feature of the intramedullary AVMs is the association with spinal aneurysms. About 20-40% of spinal intramedullary AVMs are associated with aneurysms and their presence is associated with increased risk of bleeding [7, 20].

7.2. Types

Djindjian and colleagues suggested classifying them into types based on the volume of spinal cord involved. They divided the AVMs into type I-normal volume, type II-enlarged volume and type III-intra and extramedullary AVM [12]. However, they are more simply classified by Spetzler into compact and diffuse forms [15]. The compact forms were earlier classified as glomus type and the diffuse forms were classified as juvenile AVMs. The juvenile AVMs form a distinct sub-group in that they have an embryological basis for their location. They usually arise from single or multiple somites, are usually both intra and extradural and may involve soft tissue and bone in addition to the spinal cord parenchyma. Most often they are diffuse and do not have a nidus. They may also be a manifestation of a syndromic complex such as the metameric angiomatosis (Cobb's syndrome), disseminated angiodysplasia (Osler-Weber-Rendu syndrome), Klippel-Trenaunay syndrome, or Parkes-Weber syndrome.

http://dx.doi.org/10.5772/56731

7.3. Clinical manifestations

Patients usually present in the first three decades of life, most commonly in the third decade. Hemorrhage is seen in up to 50% of patients. About 25% patients present with motor and sensory symptoms. The risk of re-bleeding in patients presenting with hemorrhage is 10% at one month and 40% at one year [22]. No sex predilection is seen in the adult population, but in childhood boys are more likely to be affected than girls. Non-hemorrhagic manifestations include back pain, radicular pain, motor/sensory deficits, sexual disturbance, sphincter disturbances and bruit. Conus AVMs, due to their location present most often with radicular pain, and involvement of the cauda equina.

Five factors contribute to the spectrum of clinical manifestations in patients with spinal AVMs.

Hemorrhage: Up to 50% of patients present with subarachnoid hemorrhage or acute medullary syndrome. These patients may present with moderate to severe backache and sudden neurologic deficit. The clinical course is often consists of progressive neurologic deficit with repeated hemorrhage. Sometimes, the patient may relate the onset of symptoms to a trivial trauma which may not be related to the neurological deficit. Spinal aneurysms located on the feeding arteries or draining veins may rupture causing acute onset neurologic deficits and/or low backache. Intracranial subarachnoid hemorrhage has also been reported due to spinal vascular malformation [21, 29].

Venous hypertension: As in intracranial AVMs, the arterialized veins have dysplastic walls and are not capable of handling high blood pressure. The resulting venous hypertension either leads to rupture of these vessels and hemorrhage or causes venous congestion and ischemia of the surrounding neural tissue due to pressure effect. Symptoms may be positional with maneuvers such as squatting or raising the leg above heart level causing increased venous congestion and exacerbation of symptoms.

Venous thrombosis: Thrombosis due to venous congestion is seen predominantly in low flow AVMs. Partial or complete thrombosis causes venous hypertension and predisposes to ischemic damage of surrounding parenchyma and hemorrhage.

Vascular steal: The phenomenon of vascular steal due to high blood flow is seen in high-flow AVMs. The AVM vessels are dysplastic and do not respond to regulatory signals. With limited ability to vasoconstrict, more blood is diverted to the AVM and the surrounding normal tissue suffers ischemic damage.

Mechanical compression: The bulky arterialized veins can cause compression of the surrounding parenchyma leading to progressive neurologic deficits. Depending upon the level where the spinal cord and nerve root are compressed, the patient may present with a combination of myelopathy and radiculopathy.

7.4. Imaging

A high index of suspicion is required to diagnose the lesions. Magnetic resonance imaging (MRI) and magnetic resonance angiography (MRA) are the first choice of investigation although angiography is the gold standard for definitive diagnosis and characterization of these lesions. MR features suggestive of vascular malformations include a serpentine pattern of low signal on T1 and T2WI (flow in dilated tortuous vessels of the arterialized coronal venous plexus), scalloped appearance on T1WI (Arterialized pial veins may focally indent the cord surface) and spinal cord signal changes due to venous congestion, myelomalacia, infarction and hemorrhage. MRA is increasingly being used for the diagnosis, localization and characterization of spinal AVMs. Mull et al reported identification of the feeding artery in 10 out of 11 patients with intradural spinal AVMs [8]. The limitations of MRA are difficulty in detection of multiple feeding vessels, low sensitivity for detection of spinal aneurysms, and inability to offer therapy in the same sitting. (Figure 5)

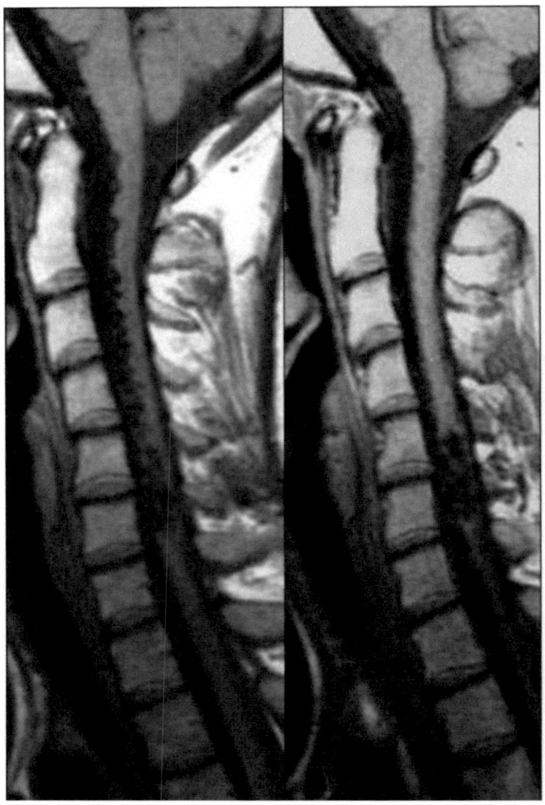

Figure 5. T1 Sagittal MRI showing serpentine "low signal" within the parenchyma of the cervical spinal cord

Digital subtraction angiography is the gold standard for diagnosis and characterization of spinal AVMs. It also offers the opportunity to treat these lesions in the same sitting. All the segmental arteries are individually catheterized on both sides to avoid missing silent lesions. The vertebral artery, thyrocervical trunk, costocervical trunk, intercostal arteries, lumbar intersegmental arteries, internal iliac arteries and sacral arteries should be visualized during the procedure. Important information to be sought on DSA includes (1) Location of AVF/AVM, feeding pedicle (2) side and site of AVF/AVM (left/right, dorsal/ventral) (3) type of fistula

http://dx.doi.org/10.5772/56731

(dural / epidural / perimedullary) (4) location of anterior spinal and posterior spinal arteries in relation to the lesion. (Figure 6)

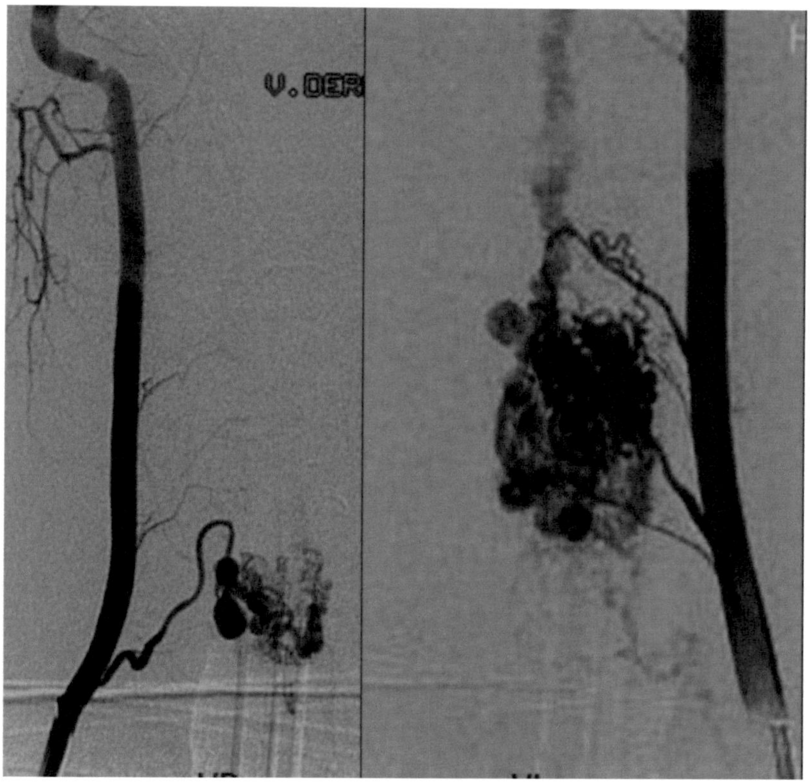

Figure 6. Spinal angiogram revealing an intramedullary AVF supplied by the vertebral artery

7.5. Treatment

The first successful surgery for spinal AVM was carried out by Elsberg in 1912. The goal of treatment is total obliteration or complete excision of the lesion. However, in some cases of juvenile AVMs, the risks associated with treatment outweigh the potential benefits from treatment. In these cases, observation may be the best choice.

There are three modalities for treatment of spinal AVMs (1) surgery (2) endovascular and (3) stereotactic radiosurgery. In some cases a combination of two modalities may have to be employed to tackle the lesion.

Surgical excision remains the gold standard for the treatment of spinal AVMs. The general neurosurgical principles involved in the excision of intracranial AVMs apply. For intramedullary lesions, a midline myelotomy is performed and the nidus is dissected carefully all around. The feeder arteries are interrupted first followed by the draining veins in the end. Juvenile AVMs are the most difficult to treat as they extend over several spinal cord segments, have multiple feeding vessels and do not have well-defined margins. Use of intraoperative SSEP and MEP monitoring, wide laminectomy and adequate exposure helps in minimizing traction and damage to the spinal cord parenchyma. Fusion may be required in a few cases if instability is caused due to facet removal.

Endovascular therapy is used either primarily or to shrink the lesion to help in surgery. Selective catheterization of feeder arteries rather than the segmental artery helps in preventing ischemia of the normal parenchyma that the segmental artery may supply. Provocative testing of radicular arteries may be undertaken via the administration of lidocaine. If corresponding deficits are noted, embolizing the corresponding feeder may not be safe. Various embolic materials that have been used include polyvinyl alcohol particles, sponge particles, balloon occlusion, liquid embolic agents such as N-butyl cyanoacrylate (NBCA), ethylene vinyl alcohol copolymer, Onyx and finally the Guglielmi Detachable Coils (GDC). Factors favoring successful endovascular occlusion include normal anterior spinal artery separate from the nidus, short distance between the feeders and the nidus, and high flow through the lesion. Occlusion of the nidus may lead to edema of the surrounding parenchyma and neurological deterioration. This is often a self-limiting condition and the patient recovers in a few weeks. Use of corticosteroids in this period may be helpful.

Although stereotactic radiosurgery (SRS) is one of the established modalities of treatment for intracranial vascular malformations, its role in the treatment of spinal vascular malformations remains investigational. Several articles have been published describing the efficacy of SRS. In one study, the authors observed significant reduction in volumes at a mean follow-up period of 27.9 months [16]. The authors concluded that long term angiographic outcome of patients is required before any treatment recommendation is made [16].

7.6. Outcome

Spetzler et al noted 68% improvement among the 27 patients who underwent surgery for spinal intramedullary AVMs and 35% improvement in patients with conus AVMs. Endovascular therapy results in successful embolization of about 63% of spinal intramedullary AVMs [1].

8. Conus medullaris AVMs

This subset of intramedullary AVMs was proposed by Spetzler in 2002 and consists of lesions at the conus medullaris with multiple feeding arteries, multiple niduses and complex venous drainage. They have multiple direct arteriovenous shunts that derive from the anterior and posterior spinal arteries and have diffuse niduses that are usually extramedullary and pial based. An intramedullary component may also be present. Because of the special location of these lesions, patients may present with both upper and lower motor neuron symptoms. (Figure 7)

http://dx.doi.org/10.5772/56731

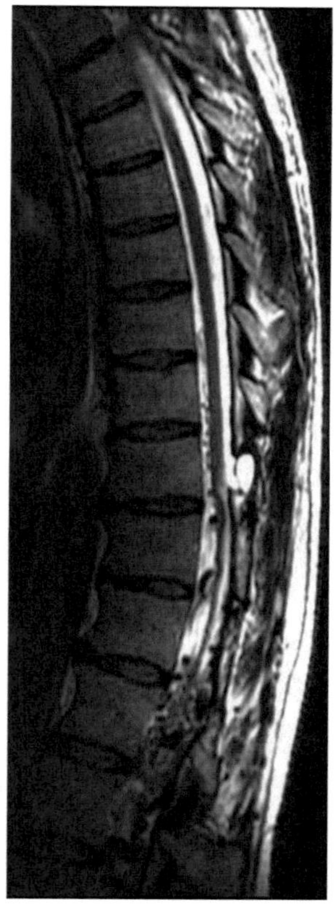

Figure 7. T2 Sagittal MRI showing tortuous vessels at the level of the conus in a male presenting with severe cauda equina syndrome.

9. Conclusion

Spinal arteriovenous lesions are a rare and diverse group of lesions that can pose challenges for clinicians both in diagnosis and treatment. Preoperative workup with quality imaging including MRI and angiogram is necessary to delineate the vascular anatomy as well as the effect on the spinal cord parenchyma. With this knowledge the proper open, endovascular, or combined treatment can be selected.

Author details

Benjamin Brown, Chiazo Amene, Shihao Zhang, Sudheer Ambekar, Hugo Cuellar and Bharat Guthikonda

LSU Health – Shreveport, LA, USA

References

[1] Biondi A, Merland JJ, Hodes JE, Pruvo JP, Reizine D. Aneurysms of spinal arteries associated with intramedullary arteriovenous malformations. I. Angiographic and clinical aspects. *AJNR Am J Neuroradiol.* 1992;13(3):913–922.

[2] Kim LJ, Spetzler RF. Classification and surgical management of spinal arteriovenous lesions: arteriovenous fistulae and arteriovenous malformations. *Neurosurgery.* 2006;59(5 Suppl 3):S195–201; discussion S3–13.

[3] Heros RC, Debrun GM, Ojemann RG, Lasjaunias PL, Naessens PJ. Direct spinal arteriovenous fistula: a new type of spinal AVM. Case report. *J. Neurosurg.* 1986;64(1): 134–139.

[4] Symon L, Kuyama H, Kendall B. Dural arteriovenous malformations of the spine. Clinical features and surgical results in 55 cases. *J. Neurosurg.* 1984;60(2):238–247.

[5] Jellema K, Tijssen CC, van Gijn J. Spinal dural arteriovenous fistulas: a congestive myelopathy that initially mimics a peripheral nerve disorder. *Brain.* 2006;129(Pt 12): 3150–3164.

[6] Niimi Y, Berenstein A, Setton A, Neophytides A. Embolization of spinal dural arteriovenous fistulae: results and follow-up. *Neurosurgery.* 1997;40(4):675–682; discussion 682–683.

[7] Biondi A, Merland JJ, Reizine D, et al. Embolization with particles in thoracic intramedullary arteriovenous malformations: long-term angiographic and clinical results. *Radiology.* 1990;177(3):651–658.

[8] Mull M, Nijenhuis RJ, Backes WH, et al. Value and limitations of contrast-enhanced MR angiography in spinal arteriovenous malformations and dural arteriovenous fistulas. *AJNR Am J Neuroradiol.* 2007;28(7):1249–1258.

[9] Krings T, Thron AK, Geibprasert S, et al. Endovascular management of spinal vascular malformations. *Neurosurg Rev.* 2010;33(1):1–9.

[10] Asai J, Hayashi T, Fujimoto T, Suzuki R. Exclusively epidural arteriovenous fistula in the cervical spine with spinal cord symptoms: case report. *Neurosurgery.* 2001;48(6): 1372–1375; discussion 1375–1376.

[11] Anson JA, Spetzler RF. Interventional neuroradiology for spinal pathology. *Clin Neurosurg.* 1992;39:388–417.

[12] Djindjian M, Djindjian R, Rey A, Hurth M, Houdart R. Intradural extramedullary spinal arterio-venous malformations fed by the anterior spinal artery. *Surg Neurol.* 1977;8(2):85–93.

[13] Mourier KL, Gobin YP, George B, Lot G, Merland JJ. Intradural perimedullary arteriovenous fistulae: results of surgical and endovascular treatment in a series of 35 cases. *Neurosurgery*. 1993;32(6):885–891; discussion 891.

[14] Barrow DL, Colohan AR, Dawson R. Intradural perimedullary arteriovenous fistulas (type IV spinal cord arteriovenous malformations). *J. Neurosurg*. 1994;81(2):221–229.

[15] Spetzler RF, Detwiler PW, Riina HA, Porter RW. Modified classification of spinal cord vascular lesions. *J. Neurosurg*. 2002;96(2 Suppl):145–156.

[16] Sinclair J, Chang SD, Gibbs IC, Adler JR Jr. Multisession CyberKnife radiosurgery for intramedullary spinal cord arteriovenous malformations. *Neurosurgery*. 2006;58(6): 1081–1089; discussion 1081–1089.

[17] Steinmetz MP, Chow MM, Krishnaney AA, et al. Outcome after the treatment of spinal dural arteriovenous fistulae: a contemporary single-institution series and meta-analysis. *Neurosurgery*. 2004;55(1):77–87; discussion 87–88.

[18] Gjertsen O, Nakstad PH, Pedersen H, Dahlberg D. Percutaneous intravertebral body embolization of a traumatic spinal epidural arteriovenous fistula with secondary perimedullary venous reflux. A case report. *Interv Neuroradiol*. 2010;16(1):97–102.

[19] Hall WA, Oldfield EH, Doppman JL. Recanalization of spinal arteriovenous malformations following embolization. *J. Neurosurg*. 1989;70(5):714–720.

[20] Rosenblum B, Oldfield EH, Doppman JL, Di Chiro G. Spinal arteriovenous malformations: a comparison of dural arteriovenous fistulas and intradural AVM's in 81 patients. *J. Neurosurg*. 1987;67(6):795–802.

[21] van Beijnum J, Straver DCG, Rinkel GJE, Klijn CJM. Spinal arteriovenous shunts presenting as intracranial subarachnoid haemorrhage. *J. Neurol*. 2007;254(8):1044–1051.

[22] da Costa L, Dehdashti AR, terBrugge KG. Spinal cord vascular shunts: spinal cord vascular malformations and dural arteriovenous fistulas. *Neurosurg Focus*. 2009;26(1):E6.

[23] Hurst RW, Kenyon LC, Lavi E, Raps EC, Marcotte P. Spinal dural arteriovenous fistula The pathology of venous hypertensive myelopathy. *Neurology*. 1995;45(7):1309–1313.

[24] Narvid J, Hetts SW, Larsen D, et al. Spinal dural arteriovenous fistulae: clinical features and long-term results. *Neurosurgery*. 2008;62(1):159–166; discussion 166–167.

[25] Bowen BC, Fraser K, Kochan JP, et al. Spinal dural arteriovenous fistulas: evaluation with MR angiography. *AJNR Am J Neuroradiol*. 1995;16(10):2029–2043.

[26] Khaldi A, Hacein-Bey L, Origitano TC. Spinal epidural arteriovenous fistula with late onset perimedullary venous hypertension after lumbar surgery: case report and discussion of the pathophysiology. *Spine*. 2009;34(21):E775–779.

[27] Silva N Jr, Januel AC, Tall P, Cognard C. Spinal epidural arteriovenous fistulas associated with progressive myelopathy. Report of four cases. *J Neurosurg Spine*. 2007;6(6):552–558.

[28] Rangel-Castilla L, Holman PJ, Krishna C, et al. Spinal extradural arteriovenous fistulas: a clinical and radiological description of different types and their novel treatment with Onyx. *J Neurosurg Spine*. 2011;15(5):541–549.

[29] Germans MR, Pennings FA, Sprengers MES, Vandertop WP. Spinal vascular malformations in non-perimesencephalic subarachnoid hemorrhage. *J. Neurol.* 2008;255(12): 1910–1915.

[30] Hirayama K, Foix C, Alajouanine T. [Subacute necrotic myelitis (Foix-Alajouanine disease) 1]. *Shinkei Kenkyu No Shimpo*. 1970;14(1):208–225.

[31] Cecchi PC, Musumeci A, Faccioli F, Bricolo A. Surgical treatment of spinal dural arterio-venous fistulae: long-term results and analysis of prognostic factors. *Acta Neurochir (Wien)*. 2008;150(6):563–570.

[32] Aminoff MJ, Logue V. The prognosis of patients with spinal vascular malformations. *Brain*. 1974;97(1):211–218.

[33] Aminoff MJ, Barnard RO, Logue V. The pathophysiology of spinal vascular malformations. *J. Neurol. Sci.* 1974;23(2):255–263.

[34] Ropper AE, Gross BA, Du R. Surgical treatment of Type I spinal dural arteriovenous fistulas. *Neurosurg Focus*. 2012;32(5):E3.

[35] Patsalides A, Santillan A, Knopman J, et al. Endovascular management of spinal dural arteriovenous fistulas. *J Neurointerv Surg*. 2011;3(1):80–84.

[36] Nichols DA, Rufenacht DA, Jack CR Jr, Forbes GS. Embolization of spinal dural arteriovenous fistula with polyvinyl alcohol particles: experience in 14 patients. *AJNR Am J Neuroradiol*. 1992;13(3):933–940.

[37] Clarke MJ, Krauss WE, Pichelmann, MA. Spinal Vascular Malormations. In: The textbook of spinal surgery. 3rd Edition.2.Philadelphia: Lippinoctt Williams and Wilkins; 2011. p. 1544-1552.

Chapter 4

Spinal Dural Arteriovenous Fistulas — Treatable Cause of Myelopathy

Antoine Nachanakian, Antonios El Helou,
Ghassan Abou Chedid and Moussa Alaywan

Additional information is available at the end of the chapter

http://dx.doi.org/10.5772/56725

1. Introduction

Arteriovenous fistula is an abnormal connection between a feeding artery and an adjacent vein. It can be congenital, acquired or created (e.g., brachial arteriovenous fistula for haemodialysis access). When it is pathological, its symptoms and diagnosis differ from one site to another in the human body.

Spinal vascular malformations (SVM) are rare diseases in comparison to vascular malformations of the brain. Spinal dural arteriovenous fistulas (SDAVFs), also known as Type I spinal arteriovenous malformations, account for 70% of spinal vascular malformations, and are the most common vascular malformations of the spinal cord and its surrounding dura mater; however, they remain relatively under-diagnosed. The majority of SDAVFs occur spontaneously, but a post-traumatic aetiology cannot be excluded in a significant proportion of them (Aghakhani N et al., 2008).

Hebold and Gaupp are credited with the first descriptions of isolated spinal cord vascular malformation in 1885 and 1888, respectively.

The first detailed clinical and pathological description of what is most likely to represent SDAVF is found in the 1926 report by Foix and Alajouanine.

Only recently did Kendall and Logue report the first case of an SDAVF as a distinct entity. Merland et al.15 illustrated the anatomical and pathological structure and location of an SDVAF in the dura mater and the intradural site of a radicular pouch. Finally, McCutcheon et al. worked on the anatomical characteristics of SDAVFs.

Diagnosis of SDAVFs is very difficult in clinical practice. In fact, symptoms are generally nonspecific.

Typically, this disease affects male patients in their 50s and 60s, causing progressive weakness of the lower limbs. Only 1% of patients are younger than 30 years of age. Most SDAVFs are solitary lesions, located between T6 and L2. Together, cervical and sacral SDAVF constitute fewer than 6% of cases. Multiple lesions in the same patient can exist, but this is rare.

2. Classification of SDAVF

According to the Spetzler classification, spinal vascular lesions can be subdivided into neoplasms, aneurysms and arteriovenous lesions. Arteriovenous lesions are further classified as arteriovenous fistulas and AVMs (Table 1).

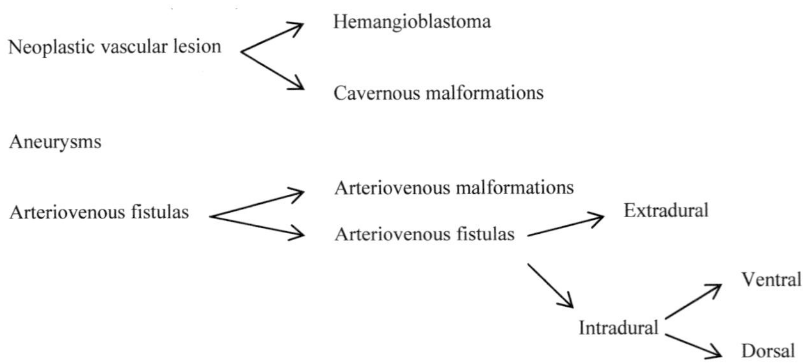

Table 1. Spetzler Classification of Spinal Vascular Malformation

Arteriovenous fistulas can either be extradural or intradural. Extradural arteriovenous fistulas have also been called epidural fistulas, and consist of a shunt between an extradural artery and a vein. Myelopathy may occasionally develop because of vascular steal (Arnaud et al., 1994a; Goyal et al., 1999).

Intradural arteriovenous fistulas are lesions causing progressive myelopathy. They may be located ventrally or dorsally. In dorsal intradural arteriovenous fistulas (SDAVF, Type I), the abnormal connection is formed between an artery and a vein at the level of a dural root sleeve with low flow, in contrast to the high-flow ventral type of fistulas. Ventral intradural arteriovenous fistulas consist of a shunt between the anterior spinal artery and an enlarged venous draining system (Djindjian et al., 1977). Type I fistulas are fed by radicular arteries and are low-pressure and low-flow vascular shunts. They are located within the dural sleeve of a nerve root and rarely entail haemorrhage; they are more commonly associated with myelopathy. Type II fistulas are located within the spinal cord itself and are true pial AVMs. They are high-pressure and high-flow shunts that are typically supplied by feeders off the anterior or posterior spinal artery or the vertebral artery. These fistulas can be associated with myelopathy or haemorrhage. Type III SDAVFs are also high-flow shunts, derived from any feeding arteries but extending both intra- and extra-durally. They are extremely rare, but also difficult to treat because of their size. Type IV SDAVFs are perimedullary fistulas, with variable flow and pressure, which can be associated with myelopathy or haemorrhage (Table 2).

Type	Characteristics	Flow
I	Direct fistula in dural sleeve of nerve root	Low pressure, low flow
II	Intramedullary	High flow, high pressure
III	Intra & extramedullary paraspinal juvenile	High pressure
IV	Intradural extramedullary direct fistula	Low to high pressure Medium to high flow

Table 2. Classification of Arteriovenous fistula.

3. Evolution from embryology to pathology

3.1. Embryology of spinal vasculature

Embryological development of the spinal vasculature occurs in four stages. The primitive segmental stage starts in the second week of gestation. 31 pairs of segmental vessels originate from paired dorsal aortas and move towards the neural tube along the developing nerve roots. Segmental vessels divide into ventral and dorsal branches and form capillary networks on the ventrolateral surface of the neural tube. These networks develop into paired primitive ventral arterial tracts, precursors of an anterior spinal artery (K. Jellema et al., 2006).

The initial stage starts in the third week. At this level, dorsal arteries anastomose with the longitudinal venous channel dorsally and ventrally.

The transitional stage follows the initial stage in the sixth week of gestation. At this stage, fusion of ventral long arterial tracts and a decrease in segmental arteries occur. At ten weeks we have the adult pattern of spinal vasculature.

Finally, the terminal stage starts after the fourth month. This stage is characterized by the maturation and increase of the tortuosity of major spinal vessels.

3.2. Anatomy of spinal vasculature

The radiculomeningeal arteries are branches of the segmental arteries (thoracic intercostal in the thoracic spine, lumbar arteries in the lumbar spine and branches of the vertebral, the deep cervical and ascending cervical arteries in the cervical spine), supplying the dura in the spinal canal, and are found at almost every spinal level. They should be distinguished from the radiculomedullary arteries, which exist only at some levels and supply the anterior and posterior spinal arteries that perfuse the spinal cord.

The venous drainage of the spinal cord does not parallel the arterial supply like the extrinsic arterial system; the extrinsic venous system has two parts: (a) longitudinal trunks, and (b) a pial plexus, termed the coronal venous plexus. The main arterial supply, the anterior spinal artery, is on the anterior surface of the cord, whereas the major venous channel is on the posterior surface, the posterior median vein. This longitudinal trunk vein has a midline location, whereas the relatively small posterior arterial trunks are off midline. In the thoraco-lumbar region, there is usually just one large anterior and one or two large posterior medullary veins, measuring up to 1.5 mm, accompanying lower thoracic or upper lumbar roots (Tadie M et al., 1985).

3.3. Pathophysiology of SDAVF

The onset in middle age suggests that SDAVF is an acquired condition, in contrast to intradural ventral fistulas or AVMs, which are assumed to be congenital abnormalities (Rosenblum et al., 1987). There are several other differences between SDAVF and AVMs. An SDAVF is never located within the spinal parenchyma. Patients with SDAVF very rarely suffer spinal haemorrhage. There are no associated vascular lesions in SDAVF. Intradural AVMs occur much more often in the cervical region (Rosenblum et al., 1987).

Aminoff and others proposed in 1974 that venous hypertension, rather than vascular steal, cord compression or haemorrhage, was the main pathophysiological factor (Aminoff et al., 1974). The shunt is most often formed within the dorsal surface of the dural root sleeve in the intervertebral foramen, where the radicular vein pierces the dura, together with one or more dural branches of the radicular artery. However, the shunt is sometimes situated along the dura between two adjacent nerve roots (Berenstein et al., 2004).

The increased pressure causes the venous system to 'arterialize', that is, the walls of intramedullary veins become thickened and tortuous. The radicular feeding artery is often a dural branch and, in a minority of cases, the medullary artery.

An increase in arterial pressure during the operation directly leads to an increase in venous pressure (Hassler et al., 1989), which may explain why some patients report that symptoms become worse after physical activity (Aminoff and Logue, 1974a; Khurana et al., 2002). Apart from the increased pressure caused by the shunt, the venous outflow may be less efficient to start with than is the case in healthy individuals (Merland et al., 1980; Thron, 2001).

The lower thoracic region has relatively fewer venous outflow channels at a segmental level than the cervical or lumbosacral region (Tadie et al., 1985). These differences in segmental outflow probably contribute to the phenomenon whereby venous congestion is transmitted in a caudo-cranial direction throughout the spinal cord, and to the fact that the first symptoms of myelopathy tend to reflect dysfunction of the lowest part of the cord, that is, the conus medullaris, even though the shunt is at the thoracic level. Possibly arteriovenous shunts are not uncommon but they become symptomatic only through congenital or environmental factors that lead to impairment of venous outflow.

The typical pathophysiologic mechanism of SDAVF is spinal cord venous hypertension, which is caused by the presence of one or a few small low-flow arteriovenous shunts between a radiculomeningeal artery and a radiculomedullary vein, usually located in the intervertebral foramen within the dura.

Thus, SDAVFs are supplied by meningeal branches that do not perfuse the spinal cord, excluding arterial steal as an associated mechanism. The SDAVF drains via a radiculomedullary vein (almost always dorsal to the cord) into the perimedullary venous system, ultimately coalescing with normal spinal cord venous drainage in a retrograde fashion. The venous drainage of the DAVF is slow and extensive along the spinal veins, and may reach the cervical spinal canal and the cranial fossa in an ascending fashion and the veins of the cauda equina in a descending fashion (Patsalides et al., 2011).

The radiculomedullary veins draining the spinal cord venous flow to the epidural space are not anatomically numerous, and SDAVF is often associated with thrombosis of radiculomedullary and epidural veins. That explains why in SDAVF a low-flow arteriovenous shunt induces high venous pressure while in congenital high-flow arteriovenous malformations venous hypertension has fewer physiopathological consequences. The pressure in the vein draining the SDAVF rises to two thirds of the mean arterial pressure, resulting in venous hypertension, which then leads to decreased arteriovenous gradient and decreased venous drainage of the spinal cord parenchyma.

Due to the slow-flow characteristics of SDAVFs, haemorrhage rarely occurs. Even though the pathophysiology of SDAVFs located on the cervical dura is similar to DAVFs in the thoracolumbar area, they may cause spinal subarachnoid haemorrhage or intracranial haemorrhage if there is venous reflux towards the brain.

3.4. Clinical presentation

Symptoms consist of myelopathy and radiculopathy and can mimic a polyradiculopathy or anterior horn cell disorder. Symptoms can progress to paraparesis or quadriparesis.

At first, almost all patients report back or leg pain with mild sensory dysfunction. Then symptoms progress slowly until diagnosis (Diaz R J et al., 2008). The mean time from the initial onset of symptoms is 15 to 23 months. In general, upper motor neuron lesion manifestations are dominant. Progressive weakness, muscle spasms, faecal incontinence, overflow urinary incontinence or urinary retention and erectile dysfunction are characteristic of myelopathy, but they are not specific to spinal dural arteriovenous fistula (Jellema K et al., 2006).

3.5. Deferential diagnosis

The differential diagnosis of nontraumatic progressive myelopathy is broad (K. Jellema, et al., 2006). The most urgent diagnoses to exclude are compressive neoplasm and infection with a spinal epidural abscess. However, other causes of increased MRI T2 cord signal are intramedullary tumours, degenerative disc disease, inflammatory and autoimmune conditions, infections, vascular disorders, and nutritional and toxic causes. Intradural tumours can be primary or metastatic and are found in the intramedullary or extramedullary space. Myelopathy due to cervical spondylosis is the most common cause of nontraumatic spastic paraparesis and quadriparesis. Lumbar canal stenosis is also common in this age group and can contribute to gait dysfunction, thus complicating the diagnosis. Myelitis can be acute (as seen in postviral infection or demyelinating myelitis) but can also be subacute to chronic conditions (e.g., AIDS myelopathy, syphilis). Inflammation of the spinal cord also occurs in several rheumatologic and connective tissue diseases, which may precede the onset of systemic symptoms by years. 16 Nutritional deficiencies should be considered in patients with gastrointestinal disease, a history of gastric bypass surgery, or a history of exposures to toxins that prevent adequate absorption of nutrients.

The time course, patient age, comorbidities, systemic symptoms, presence or absence of peripheral nervous system involvement, and localization to tracts or regions within the spinal cord can help narrow the extensive differential diagnosis for progressive myelopathy.

Many aetiologies are easily excluded by history, imaging (e.g., tumours), and serum and cerebrospinal fluid analysis (e.g., infections). However, the nonspecific features of SDAVF and frequency of both upper motor neuron signs (increased muscle tone and deep tendon reflexes) and lower motor neuron signs (flaccid weakness, depressed deep tendon reflexes) can delay diagnosis, particularly in older adults who are likely to have comorbid systemic diseases and/ or cervical spondylosis. Failure to respond to standard therapy for other causes of myelopathy should trigger further investigation.

3.6. Imaging

The essential investigations to establish the diagnosis are MRI and catheter angiography, which should be performed when a progressive myelopathy is suspected. MRI findings include hypo-intensities on T1-weighted images and hyperintensities on T2-weighted images. Increased signal intensity in the centre of the spinal cord and peripheral sparing on T2-weighted images is found in 67–100% of patients (Figure. 1) (Bowen et al., 1995; Hurst and Grossman, 2000; Luetmer et al., 2005).

In addition, abnormalities suggesting abnormal blood vessels may be seen on either the ventral or the dorsal side of the spinal cord. These 'flow void phenomena' representing tortuous and dilated veins at the dorsal surface of the spinal cord are found in 35–91% of patients (Hurst and Grossman, 2000). It seems that the flow voids are found more often, as studies are more recent, which may reflect advancement in MR techniques (Hurst and Grossman, 2000). The central hyperintense lesions are sometimes difficult to interpret, and may resemble anterior spinal artery infarction, myelitis or spinal cord neoplasms (Grandin et al., 1997), or, if slit-like, a persistent central canal (Holly and Batzdorf, 2002). Gadolinium-enhanced MRI scanning may reveal some contrast enhancement of the spinal cord (Terwey et al., 1989).

http://dx.doi.org/10.5772/56725

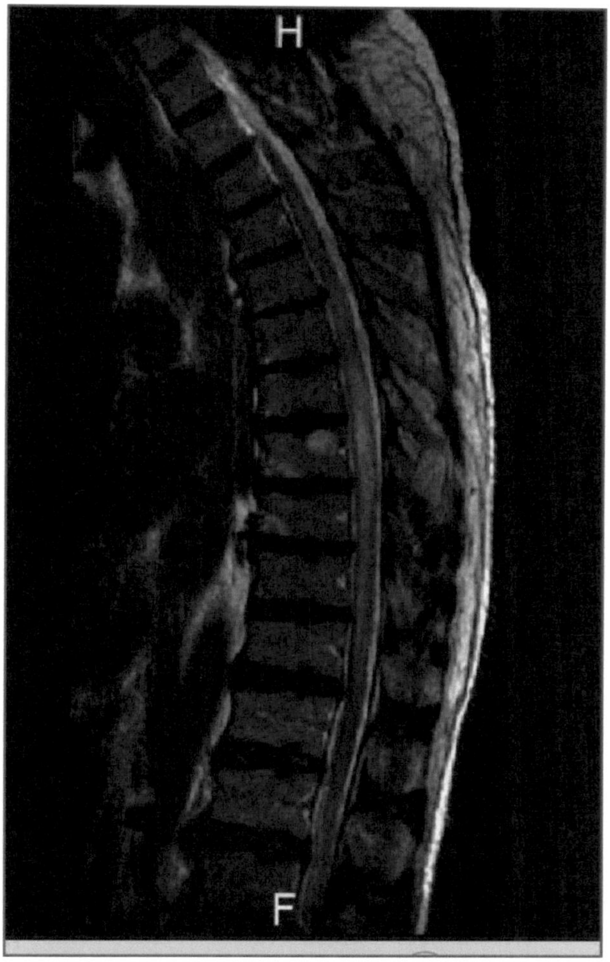

Figure 1. Sagittal T2-weighted images showing intramedullary hyperintensity.

MR angiography reveals flow in serpentine perimedullary structures (Bowen et al., 1995; Binkert et al., 1999; Mascalchi et al., 2001). MR angiography may also give an indication about the level of the SDAVF, which helps to confine the extent and duration of catheter angiography (Bowen et al., 1995; Mascalchi et al., 1999; Luetmer et al., 2005).

On the other hand, false positive MR angiography is also possible, in that normal vessels may be interpreted as being pathologically enlarged (Binkert et al., 1999; Luetmer et al., 2005).

MR TRICKS is a better tool that has improved the diagnosis of SDAVF and reduced the false positive of MR angiography (Korosec et al., 1996). First introduced by the University of Wisconsin-Madison group, time resolved imaging of contrast kinetics (TRICKS) is a method of 3D contrast-enhanced magnetic resonance angiography (MRA) providing temporal information. TRICKS combines variable rate k-space sampling, temporal interpolation of k-space views, view sharing and zero filling in the slice-encoding dimension. The interesting aspect of the method is its ability to acquire a pure arterial weighted phase; TRICKS allows ultraresolved 3D contrast-enhanced MRA without venous contamination (Albini Ricoli et al., 2007).

Before the introduction of MRI, diagnosis was often made by means of myelography (Gilbertson et al., 1995). This investigation would show an irregular, varicose dilation of the lumbar veins, sometimes giving the lumbar roots a 'postage stamp' appearance.

Catheter angiography is still the gold standard in the diagnosis of SDAVF (Figure 2). Not only the intercostal and lumbar arteries should be visualized as potential feeding arteries of an abnormal shunt, but also the median and lateral sacral artery, the deep cervical and ascending cervical arteries.

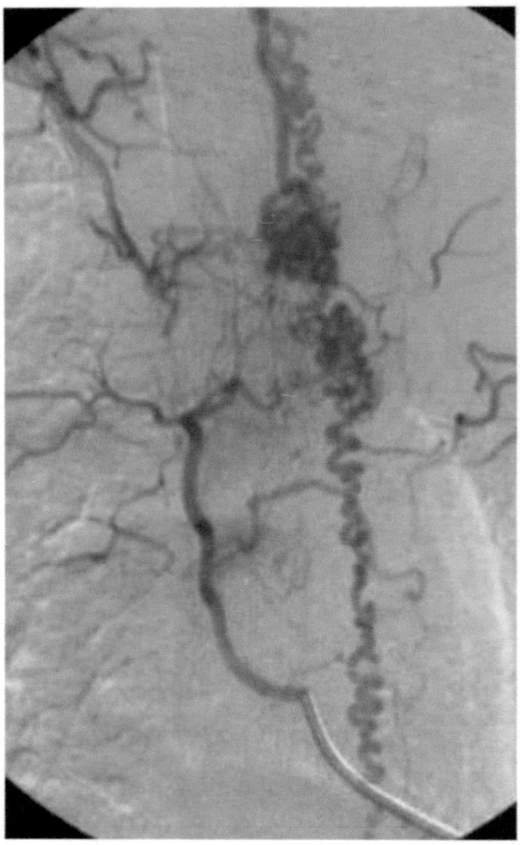

Figure 2. Spinal angiography illustrating a SDAVF fed by right Th11 radicular artery with tortuous draining veins.

The angioarchitecture of the fistula should be thoroughly investigated, especially with regard to the question of whether the arterial feeder is a dural branch or a segmental medullary artery, which also contributes to the anterior spinal artery. In the latter case, endovascular treatment is not possible, because infarction of the spinal cord is likely to occur. Furthermore, it is essential to identify the artery of Adamkiewicz, because the fistula may originate from this important tributary to the anterior spinal artery.

4. Decision making and management

4.1. Diagnostic criteria

The typical patient where SDAVF is suspected is aged 40–80 and shows a gradual onset of slowly progressive or stepwise worsening myelopathy characterized by lower-extremity weakness, sensory loss to pinprick and light touch, and late development of bowel and bladder dysfunction. Pre-operative imaging is mandatory.

MR imaging is an initial diagnostic tool. MRI assesses the level of the suspected SDAVF, shown by the flow void and the tortuosity of the vessels in addition to intramedullary hyper signal on a T2-weighted image. MRA can play a valuable role in confirming the diagnosis and targeting conventional catheter angiography.

All patients with confirmed or suspected SDAVF are evaluated by spinal angiography (Figure 3). After confirming the diagnosis, a joint decision is taken by the neurosurgery team and endovascular neuroradiology about the method of treatment.

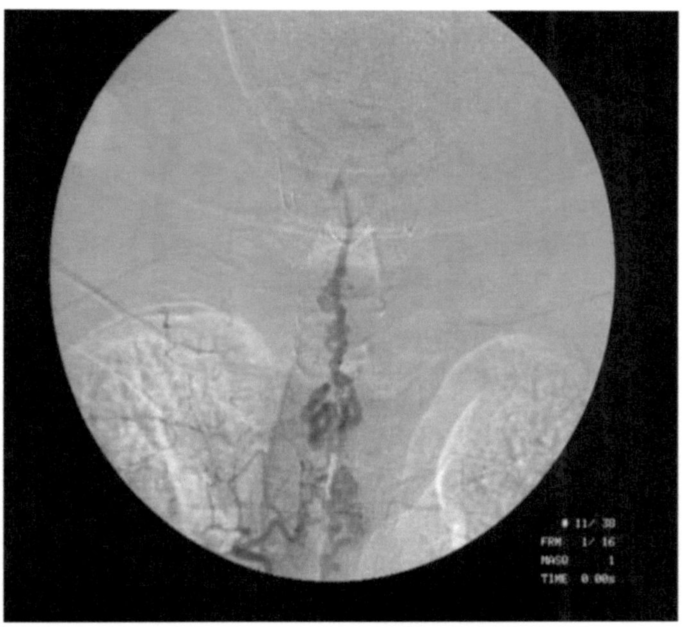

Figure 3. Spinal angiography of the left Th6 radicular artery showing SDAVF with tortuous veins extending superior to the cervico-thoracic junction level.

4.2. Indication for surgical treatment

Treatment for SDAVFs must be performed as soon as possible and may be surgical or endovascular, as both are safe and effective. Microsurgical treatment was considered the gold standard for many years but recent technical advances in endovascular surgery have made endovascular treatments an option. As with all inherent disease processes of the spinal cord, post-operative function is highly related to pre-operative presentation, and maximum functional results are obtained in patients treated early, before advanced deterioration has taken place.

4.3. Surgery

4.3.1. Pre-operative work up

All patients admitted to neurosurgery wards are clinically evaluated the day before the procedure. A full neurological examination is performed evaluating the motor, sensory, and deep tendon reflexes, as well as the gait. In addition, clinical urological evaluation and, when needed, urodynamic studies are carried out.

4.3.2. Operative procedure

The procedure is carried out under general anaesthesia. All patients are operated in a prone position, with the thoracolumbar spine segment in neutral to a slightly kyphotic position, avoiding hyperlordosis.

Intra-operative motor-evoked potential monitoring is used in all procedures with continuous observation by the neurologist until the end of the procedure.

The level of the procedure is localized after positioning under fluoroscopy. Midline vertical skin incision is carried out. The subcutaneous layer and the paraspinal muscles are dissected until the articular facets are identified.

A two-level laminectomy is carried out. A median longitudinal dural incision is performed, exposing the intradural nerve root, initial segments of draining vein and several millimetres of the feeding radicular artery (Figure 4). Intra-operative Doppler control is performed upon identification of the fistula revealing an arterial spectrum on the redundant dorsal medullary veins. After the clipping of the feeder of the arteriovenous shunt by a temporary clamp, the intra-operative monitoring documents a complete disappearance of the arterial spectrum and the reappearance of the venous pattern. In addition, the motor-evoked potential is monitored and controlled twice, at a five-minute interval. If no changes are observed in the physiological studies, the fistula is obliterated at the artery vein connection with two small permanent vascular clips. Then, it is coagulated (Figure 5).

Dural closure is performed with fascia-latta auto graft using a tight continuous running suture method. Some trials for synthetic dural graft fail due to a high rate of post-operative CSF leak.

http://dx.doi.org/10.5772/56725

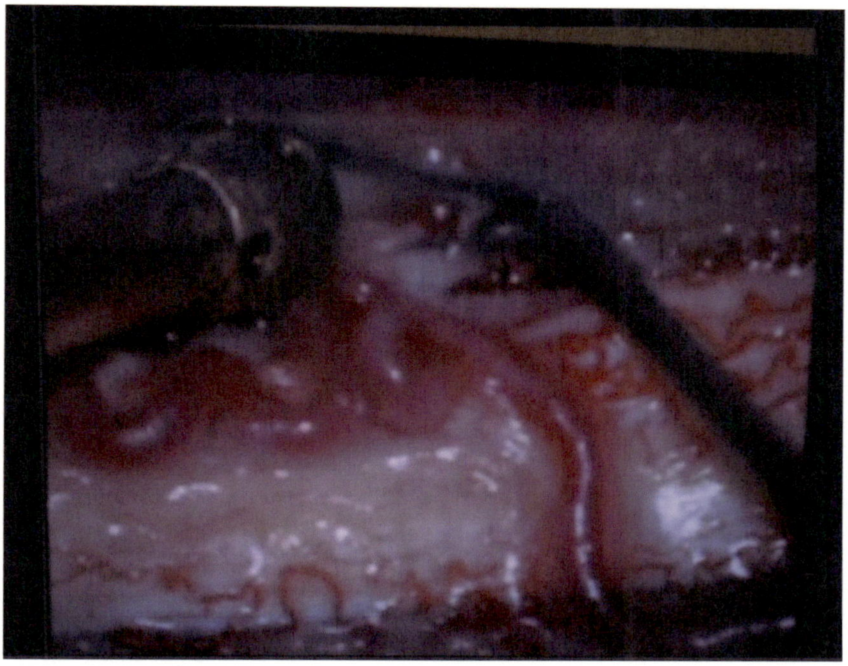

Figure 4. Pre-operative findings showing tortuous veins with artery under suction tip accompanying the nerve root beneath the spatula.

4.3.3. Post-operative care

The patient is kept in a completely supine position to avoid CSF leak and is out of bed 48 hours after surgery. Routine laboratory tests are carried out on day 1. Steroids are applied post-operatively in high dosages (Methylprednisolone, 1g every 24 hours; or Dexamethasone, 8mg every 8 hours), and this regime is continued with progressive tapering over two weeks, with a shift to oral medication in 72 hours. No imaging is ordered in the immediate post-op period, unless there is a clinical deterioration. A control spine MRI with angiography MR is carried out six months after the operation.

4.3.4. Long-term results

Overall improvement was noted in surgically treated patients, and to a considerable degree of satisfaction in approximately 75% of patients. Motor strength and gait improvement were superior to bladder function (Ropper A E et al., 2012). Deterioration of the previous neurological status was found in less than 10% of cases; persistence of stable status was found in 10–15% of the operated patients (Schick U et al., 2003, Song JK et al., 2001).

Post-operative neurological improvement progressively increased during the next three months. Patients achieved maximum improvement after an average period of six months. The prominent characteristic of this surgery is a low level of post-operative pain.

Motor and gait dysfunction improved more than sensory and bladder dysfunction with time.

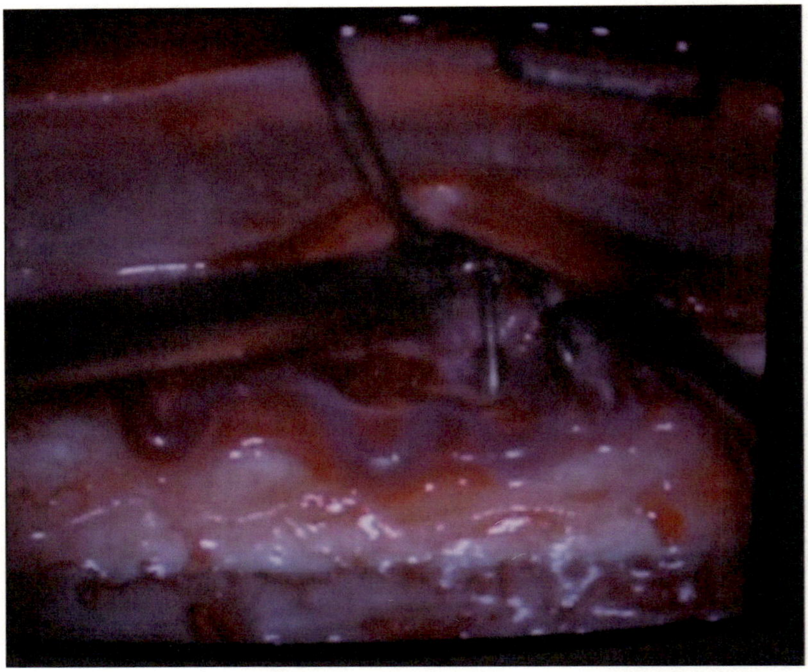

Figure 5. Pre-operative finding after clipping of the feeding artery. The image shows early shrinkage of the arterialized veins.

4.3.5. Complications

In general, this procedure is well tolerated. The overall rate of complications is between 1 and 5%. Two kinds of complications exist: the early and the delayed (Schick U et al., 2003, Song JK et al., 2001 and Ropper A E et al., 2012).

Early complications include CSF leak, infection, haematoma, and neurological sequelae.

Delayed complications depend on obliteration rate, which is around 98% in surgical patients.

4.4. Endovascular treatment

Endovascular therapy is less invasive than microsurgery, and allows both diagnosis and treatment in a single session (Park S B et al., 2008); however, more than one session may be necessary for some patients.

The ability to definitively treat spinal DAVFs using endovascular embolization has significantly improved over the last several decades. Overall rates of definitive embolization of spinal DAVFs have ranged between 25 and 100%, depending in part on the embolic agent used and the use of variable stiffness microcatheters. The majority of recent studies in which N-butyl cyanoacrylate or other liquid embolic agents were used have reported success rates of 70–90% (Sivakumar W et al., 2009). Although endovascular therapy is potentially less invasive and associated with less morbidity and earlier mobilization than surgery, endovascular therapy has been associated with a lower initial success rate and higher rate of recurrence than microsurgical therapy (Van Dijk JM et al., 2002). Several factors need to be considered when selecting endovascular therapy for the treatment of spinal DAVF. A spinal DAVF usually consists of multiple dural arterial vessels with a single draining vein. Thus, occlusion of a feeding arterial vessel may lead to recanalization or collateral development in the early post-operative period (McCutcheon IE et al., 1996). Another important consideration is the identification of patients with conditions that would make them unsuitable for endovascular therapy. Embolization therapy may not be feasible if the arterial feeder is too small to catheterize and arterial damage due to catheter manipulation is likely, as in patients with severe arteriosclerosis, or if the anterior spinal artery, the Adamkiewicz and feeding artery of the fistula originate from the same segmental artery (Thron A, 2001).

Detachable coils, silk sutures, polyvinyl alcohol (PVA), and n-butyl-2-cyanoacrylate (NBCA) have been used as embolic agents for endovascular management of DAVFs.

The use of liquid embolization material is imperative to prevent recanalization, while the use of particle embolization (polyvinyl alcohol, embospheres and gel foam) is not indicated because of its high recanalization rates. At first, N-butyl cyanoacrylate (NBCA) was often used.

Endovascular embolization of SDAVF using NBCA has a high success rate (Warakaulle DR et al., 2003). It is referred to as glue, being an extremely effective liquid acrylic polymer that polymerizes when it comes into contact with an ionic medium such as blood. NBCA is diluted with ethiodized oil to render it radiopaque and visible during the embolization. Transarterial *NBCA* embolization is highly operator-dependent because the glue quickly polymerizes, often leading to inadequate filling of the proximal draining vein. Complete filling of the proximal vein is a critical component for definitive endovascular cure of these lesions.

At present, the Onyx is used, which is a new liquid embolic agent, a mixture of ethylene-vinyl alcohol copolymer and dimethyl sulfoxide (DMSO). While DMSO diffuses under aqueous conditions the ethylene-vinyl alcohol copolymer precipitates and mechanically occludes the feeding vessels, whose viscosity makes it suitable for treatment of spinal DAVF, where penetration into the proximal radicular vein is required (Carlson AP et al., 2007; Ross et al., 2012). Contrary to NBCA, Onyx does not adhere to the biological surfaces, which allows for slow delivery and improved penetration of the nidus (Nogueira RG et al., 2009).

4.4.1. Endovascular technique

The procedure is carried out under general anaesthesia in an interventional radiology room. The patient is in a supine position. The right femoral crease is prepared for puncture.

Neurophysiological monitoring allows a warning for the neuroradiologist of impending irreversible neurological damage so that action may be taken for the prompt restoration of adequate spinal cord perfusion. Muscle motor-evoked potentials reflect spinal cord perfusion in the anterior spinal artery territory better than somatosensory-evoked potentials (SEPs). Although rarely used, motor-evoked potentials make the procedure safer (Sala F et al., 2001).

After recording baseline SEPs and MEPs, 50 mg of sodium amytal is injected through the microcatheter at the position of the intended embolization, followed by assessment of SEPs and MEPs. If no changes have occurred, 40 mg of lidocaine is then injected, followed by recording of SEPs and MEPs. If no changes are noted again, embolization is performed (Niimi et al., 2000). If there is any change in either the SEPs or the MEPs, NBCA embolization is not performed from that catheter position.

After delivery of the embolization material, DMSO leaks from the embolus allowing for Onyx to precipitate into the vessel lumen. (Figure 6).

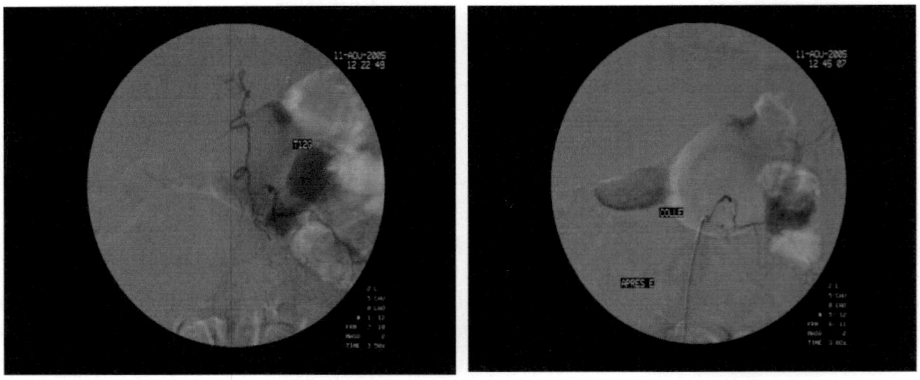

Figure 6. Left: Arteriography of SDAVF pre embolization. Right: Arteriography of the same patient post embolization.

4.4.2. Post-procedure care

The patient is transferred to a regular ward after the embolization procedure. The post-operative steroid protocol is identical to the one used in the microsurgery technique (high-dose steroids for the first two days, then progressive tapering after a shift to per os intake over two weeks).

The patients ambulate on the first day post-embolization and can be discharged on day 2. Regular clinical follow-ups are carried out one, three and six months after the procedure. A new spinal angiography is ordered six months after the endovascular procedure.

4.4.3. Complications

The risk of inadvertent embolization of arteries feeding normal tissue is high, and precise positioning of the delivery microcatheter as close as possible to the arteriovenous lesion is an important manoeuvre to prevent embolization of normal tissue. To prevent polymerization in the delivery catheter or prematurely in the vasculature, the microcatheter must first be thoroughly flushed. For NBCA solution after mixing with radiopaque solution, the microcatheter is flushed with 10–15 ml of 5% dextrose solution. On the other hand, the use of Onyx injection necessitates microcatheter flushing with saline solution to fill the dead space estimated for 0.5 to 1 ml.

The recanalization rate in all serious cases is 15–20% (Song et al., 2001; Hall WA et al., 1989). The bleeding rate and/or embolization of inadequate arteries differed between serious and other cases, fluctuating between 0 and 4% (Schick U and Hassler W, 2003; Steinmetz MP et al. 2004).

5. Institution experience

Our experience is based on 16 cases of SDAVF treated from January 2003 to March 2012. Eleven cases were managed surgically, whereas five were treated by endovascular embolization. This decision was based on age, clinical symptoms, and the level of the fistula.

87.5% of our patients were male. The mean age was 65 years. Three cases were in the lumbar level, one in the sacral and 12 in the thoracic region. Fifteen cases had a radicular artery feeder, one had an intercostal feeder and one was identified incidentally during an interlaminar approach for a herniated disc.

We recorded three cases of radiculopathy in our series. All other patients showing signs of progressive myelopathy worsened over long-term periods.

In our institution, patients are admitted for 24 hours before the day of the procedure, and as early as possible after initial diagnosis.

In the pre-operative period, the patient is treated with anti-platelets and other anti-coagulation agents for five days. Only LMWH can be tolerated up to 12 hours before the procedure.

If the treatment decided upon is surgical, patients ambulate 48 hours after the procedure; those treated by endovascular embolization ambulate within 24 hours of the procedure.

All patients are assessed using the Aminoff-Logue disability scale in the pre-op and post-op periods.

Usually, patients have regular follow-ups at one, three and 12 months.

Patients at first reported an improvement of their radicular pain, with a mean reduction of 4.3/10 on visual analogue scale (VAS) (0: absent pain, to 10: severe intolerable pain necessitating intra-venous treatment). In the pre-operative period, radicular pain when extant had a mean score of 7.8/10 on VAS; in the immediate post-op period, the pain was 3.4/10 on VAS.

We did not observe any complications in the surgically treated patients, although recanalization occurred in one of the patients treated by embolization. No bleeding or embolization at other sites was observed.

6. Conclusion

With progressive myelopathy of unknown origin in a middle-aged patient, SDAVF must always be considered. Magnetic resonance imaging, especially the new 3T generation, is a good initial tool to identify the tortuous veins around the spinal cord and spinal cord oedema, especially on T2WI. Spinal catheter angiography remains the gold standard for diagnosis and identification of the site of the fistula. These vascular malformations can be treated either by endovascular embolization or surgical clipping, keeping in mind that the latter has a higher occlusion rate.

Author details

Antoine Nachanakian, Antonios El Helou, Ghassan Abou Chedid and Moussa Alaywan

Division of Neurosurgery and Endovascular Neuroradiology, Saint George Hospital University Medical Center, Balamand University, Lebanon

References

[1] Aghakhani N, Parker F, David P, et al. Curable cause of paraplegia: spinal dural arteriovenous fistulae. Stroke 2008; 39: 2756e9.

[2] Albini Riccioli L, Marliani A F, Ghedin P, Agati R, and Leonardi M. CE-MR Angiography at 3.0 T Magnetic Field in the Study of Spinal Dural Arteriovenous Fistula. Interv Neuroradiol 2007; 13(1): 13–18.

[3] Aminoff MJ, Barnard RO, Logue V. The pathophysiology of spinal vascular malformations. J Neurol Sci 1974; 23: 255–63.

[4] Arnaud O, Pelletier J, Dalecky A, Cherif AA, Azulay JP, Salamon G, et al. Spinal dural fistula with peri-medullar venous drainage. Rev Neurol (Paris) 1994b; 150: 713–20.

[5] Patsalides A, Santillan A, Knopman J, Tsiouris AJ, Riina HA, Gobin YP. Endovascular management of spinal dural arteriovenous fistulas. J NeuroIntervent Surg 2011; 3: 80e84. doi:10.1136/jnis.2010.003178.

[6] Berenstein A, Lasjaunias P, Ter Brugge KG. editors. Surgical neuroangiography 2.2. Berlin: Springer; 2004.

[7] Binkert CA, Kollias SS, Valavanis A. Spinal cord vascular disease: characterization with fast three-dimensional contrast-enhanced MR angiography. AJNR Am J Neuroradiol 1999; 20: 1785–93.

[8] Bowen BC, Fraser K, Kochan JP, Pattany PM, Green BA, Quencer RM. Spinal dural arteriovenous fistulas: evaluation with MR angiography. AJNR Am J Neuroradiol 1995; 16: 2029.

[9] Carlson AP, Taylor CL, Yonas H. Treatment of dural arteriovenous fistula using ethylene vinyl alcohol (onyx) arterial embolization as the primary modality: Short-term results. J Neurosurg 2007; 107: 1120-5.

[10] Diaz RJ and Wong JH. Spinal dural arteriovenous fistula: a treatable cause of myelopathy. CMAJ 2008; 178(10): 1286–1288.

[11] Djindjian M, Djindjian R, Rey A, Hurth M, Houdart R. Intradural extramedullary spinal arterio-venous malformations fed by the anterior spinal artery. Surg Neurol 1977; 8: 85–93.

[12] Eskandar EN, Borges LF, Budzik RF Jr, et al. Spinal dural arteriovenous fistulas: experience with endovascular and surgical therapy. J Neurosurg 2002; 96(2 Suppl): 162e7.

[13] Gilbertson JR, Miller GM, Goldman MS, Marsh WR. Spinal dural arteriovenous fistulas: MR and myelographic findings. AJNR Am J Neuroradiol 1995; 16: 2049–57.

[14] Goyal M, Willinsky R, Montanera W, Ter Brugge K. Paravertebral arteriovenous malformations with epidural drainage: clinical spectrum, imaging features, and results of treatment. AJNR Am J Neuroradiol 1999; 20: 749–55.

[15] Grandin C, Duprez T, Stroobandt G, Laterre EC, Mathurin P. Spinal dural arterio-venous fistula: an underdiagnosed disease? Acta Neurol Belg 1997; 97: 17–21.

[16] Guo LM, Zhou HY, Xu JW, et al. Dural arteriovenous fistula at the foramen magnum presenting with subarachnoid hemorrhage: case reports and literature review. Eur J Neurol 2010; 17:684e91.

[17] Hall WA, Oldfield EH, Doppman JL. Recanalization of spinal arteriovenous malformations following embolization. J Neurosurg. 1989; 70:714–720.

[18] Hassler W, Thron A. Flow velocity and pressure measurements in spinal dural arteriovenous fistulas. Neurosurg Rev 1994; 17: 29–36.

[19] Hurst RW, Grossman RI. Peripheral spinal cord hypointensity on T2-weighted MR images: a reliable imaging sign of venous hypertensive myelopathy. AJNR Am J Neuroradiol 2000; 21: 781–6.

[20] Holly LT, Batzdorf U. Slitlike syrinx cavities: a persistent central canal. J Neurosurg 2002; 97: 161–5.

[21] Jellema K, Sluzewski M, van Rooij WJ, et al. Embolization of spinal dural arteriovenous fistulas: importance of occlusion of the draining vein. J Neurosurg Spine 2005; 2: 580e3.

[22] Jellema K, Tijssen CC, van Gijn J. Spinal dural arteriovenous fistulas: a congestive myelopathy that initially mimics a peripheral nerve disorder. Brain 2006; 129: 3150–64.

[23] Khurana VG, Perez-Terzic CM, Petersen RC, Krauss WE. Singing paraplegia: a distinctive manifestation of a spinal dural arteriovenous fistula. Neurology 2002; 58: 1279–81.

[24] Korosec FR, Frayne R, et al. Time-resolved contrast-enhanced 3D MR angiography. Magn Reson Med. 1996; 36: 345–351.

[25] Luetmer PH, Lane JI, Gilbertson JR, Bernstein MA, Huston J III, Atkinson JL. Preangiographic evaluation of spinal dural arteriovenous fistulas with elliptic centric contrast-enhanced MR angiography and effect on radiation

[26] dose and volume of iodinated contrast material. AJNR Am J Neuroradiol 2005; 26: 711–8.

[27] Mascalchi M, Ferrito G, Quilici N, Mangiafico S, Cosottini M, Cellerini M, et al. Spinal vascular malformations: MR angiography after treatment. Radiology 2001; 219: 346–53.

[28] Merland JJ, Riche MC, Chiras J. Intraspinal extramedullary arteriovenous fistulae draining into the medullary veins. J Neuroradiol 1980; 7: 271e320.

[29] Merland JJ, Assouline E, Rufenacht D, Guimaraens L, Laurent A. Dural spinal arteriovenous fistulae draining into medullary veins: clinical and radiological results of treatment (embolization and surgery) in 56 cases. Excerpta Med Int Congr Ser 1986; 698: 283–9.

[30] McCutcheon IE, Doppman JL, Oldfield EH. Microvascular anatomy of dural arteriovenous abnormalities of the spine: a microangiographic study. J Neurosurg 1996; 84: 215–220.

[31] Niimi Y, Sala F, Deletis V, Berenstein A. Provocative Testing for Embolization of Spinal Cord AVMs. Interv Neuroradiol. 2000; 30; 6 Suppl 1: 191–4.

[32] Nogueira RG, Dabus G, Rabinov JD, Ogilvy CS, Hirsch JA, Pryor JC. Onyx embolization for the treatment of spinal dural arteriovenous fistulae: Initial experience with long-term follow-up: Technical case report. Neurosurgery 2009; 64: E197–8.

[33] Park SB, Han MH, Jahng TA, Kwon BJ, and Chung CK. Spinal Dural Arteriovenous Fistulas: Clinical Experience with Endovascular Treatment as a Primary Therapeutic Modality. J Korean Neurosurg Soc 2008; 44(6): 364–369.

[34] Ropper AE, Gross BA, Du R. Surgical Treatment of Type I Spinal Dural Arteriovenous Fistulas. Neurosurg Focus 2012; 32(5): e3

[35] Rosenblum B, Oldfield EH, Doppman JL, Di Chiro G. Spinal arteriovenous malformations: a comparison of dural arteriovenous fistulas and intradural AVMs in 81 patients. J Neurosurg 1987; 67: 795–802

[36] Ross C, Puffer RC, Daniels DJ, Kallmes DF, Cloft HJ, Lanzino G. Curative Onyx Embolization of Tentorial Dural Arteriovenous Fistulas. Neurosurg Focus. 2012; 32(5): e4

[37] Sala F, Niimi Y, Berenstein A, Deletis V. Neuroprotective role of neurophysiological monitoring during endovascular procedures in the spinal cord. Ann N Y Acad Sci 2001; 939: 126–36.

[38] Schaat TJ, Salzman KL, Stevens EA. Sacral origin of a spinal dural arteriovenous fistula: case report and review. Spine (Phila Pa 1976) 2002; 27: 893e7.

[39] Schick U and Hassler W. Treatment and outcome of spinal dural arteriovenous fistulas. Eur Spine J. 2003; 12(4): 350–355.

[40] Sivakumar W, Zada G, Yashar P, Giannotta SL, Teitelbaum G, Larsen DW. Endovascular management of spinal dural arteriovenous fistulas. A review. Neurosurg Focus 2009; 26(5): E15.

[41] Song JK, Vinuela F, Gobin YP, Duckwiler GR, Murayama Y, Kureshi I, Frazee JG, Martin NA. Surgical and endovascular treatment of spinal dural arteriovenous fistulas: long-term disability assessment and prognostic factors. J Neurosurg. 2001; 94(2 Suppl): 199–204.

[42] Steinmetz MP, Chow MM, Krishnaney AA, Andrews-Hinders D, Benzel EC, Masaryk TJ, Mayberg MR, Rasmussen PA. Outcome after the treatment of spinal dural arteriovenous fistulae: a contemporary single-institution series and meta-analysis. Neurosurgery 2004; 55(1): 77–87.

[43] Tadie M, Hemet J, Freger P, Clavier E, Creissard P. Morphological and functional anatomy of spinal cord veins. J Neuroradiol 1985; 12: 3–20.

[44] Thron A. Spinal dural arteriovenous fistulas. Radiologe 2001; 41: 955–60.

[45] Terwey B, Becker H, Thron AK, Vahldiek G. Gadolinium-DTPA enhanced MR imaging of spinal dural arteriovenous fistulas. J Comput Assist Tomogr 1989; 13: 30–7.

[46] Thron A. Spinal dural arteriovenous fistulas. Radiologe 2001; 41: 955–960.

[47] Tsai LK, Jeng JS, Liu HM, Wang HJ, Yip PK. Intracranial dural arteriovenous fistulas with or without cerebral sinus thrombosis: analysis of 69 patients. J Neurol Neurosurg Psychiatry 2004; 75: 1639–41.

[48] Van Dijk JM, Ter Brugge KG, Willinsky RA, Farb RI, Wallace MC. Multidisciplinary management of spinal dural arteriovenous fistulas: clinical presentation and long-term follow-up in 49 patients. Stroke 2002; 33: 1578–1583

[49] Warakaulle DR, Aviv RI, Niemann D, Molyneux AJ, Byrne JV, Teddy P. Embolisation of spinal dural arteriovenous fistulae with Onyx. Neuroradiology 2003; 45(2): 110–2.

Chapter 5

Spinal Arteriovenous Fistulas and Arteriovenous Malformations – Complicated Vasculature and Surgical Imaging

Shinji Yamamoto and Phyo Kim

Additional information is available at the end of the chapter

http://dx.doi.org/10.5772/56367

1. Introduction

Spinal arteriovenous shunts (AV shunts; including spinal AV fistulas and AV malformations) are heterogeneous entities that can render devastating neurological sequelae by hemorrhage (hematomyelia, subarachnoid hemorrhage, and subdural/epidural hematoma), venous congestion, mass effect, and vascular steal [1-5]. These lesions have been challenging entities to treat because of their complicated vasculature and the high-vulnerability of the spinal cord.

In the absence of accumulated knowledge of the pathophysiology of each entity, early classifications were based on the anatomical characteristics, which could be confusing [6-10]. With evolution of imaging technology such as various MR imaging, CT angiography and selective spinal angiography, ability to examine the angioarchitecture of these lesions has improved significantly. In addition, intraoperative diagnostic modalities have been developed that aid in open microsurgery before, during, and after the resection of these lesions. Increased knowledge of the angioarchitecture and pathophysiology of spinal AV shunts has led to the development of a multidisciplinary approach to these lesions.

This article, after the description of spinal vessel anatomy and some practical classification schemes, follows the recent advancement of spinal vascular imagings and intraoperative diagnostic tools for open microsurgery, which are indispensable for the effective treatment of spinal complex vascular lesions.

2. Spinal vasculature

To understand the pathophysiology of spinal AV shunts, a profound knowledge of spinal vessel anatomy is indispensable.

2.1. Segmental spinal arteries

Blood supply to a metamere that consists of vertebral body, paraspinal muscles, dura, nerve root and spinal cord is derived from segmental arteries, that are present in the fetus for each metameres (the 31 spinal segments). The segmental arteries potentially supply all the tissues on one side of a given metamere. Each metamere is centered at the level of the intervertebral disc, and each vertebra is therefore supplied by two consecutive segmental arteries on each side which build sufficient transverse and longitudinal anastomoses. These extra- and intraspinal anastomoses provide excellent collateral circulation, and protect the spinal cord against ischemia. The segmental arteries course along the vertebral body posteriorly, supplying blood to the vertebral body through perforating arteries. While the muscular branches run further posteriorly to the segmental muscles, the spinal branches enter the spinal canal through the intervertebral foramen and divide into the following three branches: the anterior and posterior branches which supply blood to the bony structure, and the radicular artery which supply blood to the dura and the nerve tissue at every segmental level [11].

Lasjanias *et al.* proposed a useful classification of the radicular arteries based on their region of supply, i.e., radicular, radiculopial and radiculomedullary [12]. The first type of radicular artery is a small branch, present at every segmental level, whose supply is restricted to the dura and the nerve root. The second type of radiculopial artery supplies blood to the nerve root and superficial pial system, including the posterior spinal arteries. The third type of radiculomedullary artery supplies the nerve root, superficial pial system, and the anterior spinal artery. Although the anterior and posterior spinal arteries are connected with the superficial pial collateral system, this classification provides a reasonable basis for planning treatment. In fact, a given segmental artery may connect to both the anterior and posterior arteries. These three types of the radicular artery are classified in terms of their contribution to each spinal artery.

Whereas each radicular artery supplies blood to the spinal cord in the embryo, the number of radicular arteries supplying the spinal cord decreases following a transformation and fusion in the postnatal life [13]. At certain segmental levels, the radicular artery has a persistent supply to the spinal cord that reaches either the anterior surface via the ventral nerve root or the posterolateral surface via the dorsal nerve root. Between two to 14, (on average, 6), radiculomedullary arteries persist as the result of this ontogenic reduction in feeding arteries. The radiculopial arteries are also reduced to fewer than 11 and 16 arteries.

2.2. Arteries of the spinal cord

The anterior spinal artery, with a diameter of 0.2–1.0 mm, traverses along the anterior median sulcus and typically originates from the intracranial portion of the vertebral arteries. The posterior spinal arteries, with a diameter of 0.1–0.4 mm, originate from the preatlantal part of the vertebral artery or from the posterior inferior cerebellar artery (PICA). These arteries course from the cervical spine to the conus medullaris but are not capable of feeding the entire spinal cord. They are reinforced at various segmental levels by the radiculomedullary/radiculopial arteries [12]. The blood flow derived from these segmental arteries may be both caudocranial and craniocaudal. The most well-known radiculomedullary artery is the artery of Adamkiewicz (arteria radicularis magna), which arises close to the thoracolumbar enlargement. On the entire surface of the cord, both anterior/posterior spinal arteries anastomose via an extensive pial network (vasacorona). At the level of the conus medullaris, the posterior spinal arteries are connected to the anterior spinal artery through the anastomotic semicircles [11].

The intrinsic arteries of the spinal cord can be divided into two perforating systems–the sulcal (central, sulco-commissural) arteries originate from the anterior spinal artery, and the perforating rami arise from the vasacorona. Sulcal arteries, with a diameter of 0.1–0.25mm, are centrifugal and supply the largest part of the gray matter. They penetrate into the parenchyma through the anterior median fissure, course to one side of the cord and branch mainly within the gray matter. These arteries can anastomose via the transmedullary arteries with the deep perforating arteries from the vasacorona. Numerous perforating rami, with a diameter of up to 0.05 mm, penetrate the white matter, forming a centripetal system [11].

2.3. Spinal venous system

The venous drainage from the spinal cord comprises the small superficial pial veins that open into the superficial longitudinal veins. On the surface of the cord, blood accumulates in essentially two longitudinal veins–the anterior and posterior spinal veins. The anterior spinal vein is located under the anterior spinal artery in the subpial space. The posterior spinal vein, located in the subarachnoid space perimedullarily, takes a course independent of the posterior spinal arteries. The perimedullary venous system is more variable in course, size, and localization than the arterial system. Intraparenchymal transmedullary venous anastomoses may be present; these midline anastomoses, 0.3–0.7mm in diameter, connect the anterior and posterior spinal veins while receiving no tributaries from the intrinsic spinal cord veins [14].

The perimedullary venous collectors drain into the epidural venous plexus through the radicular veins. The transition from the perimedullary vein to the radicular vein forms a hairpin course, similar to the arterial configuration. Drainage of blood from the spinal cord is directed to the epidural plexus without retrograde flow. Though there is no valve structure in the spinal venous plexus, the nature of this reflux-impending mechanism is a matter of dispute. Some histological studies showed that the anatomical features act as an antireflux device–a substantial narrowing and bending of the vessels at its transdural course [14, 15]. These characteristics result either from the close proximity of a nerve root or from the presence of a bulge of dural collagenous fibers with a glomus-like appearance, which were supposed to act an antireflux mechanism physiologically.

The epidural venous plexus extends as a continuous system from the sacrum to the skull base and is located within the fatty and fibrous tissues of the epidural space. This valveless system is connected with the azygos/hemiazygos venous systems in the thoracolumbar region, and with the vertebral and deep cervical veins in the cervical region.

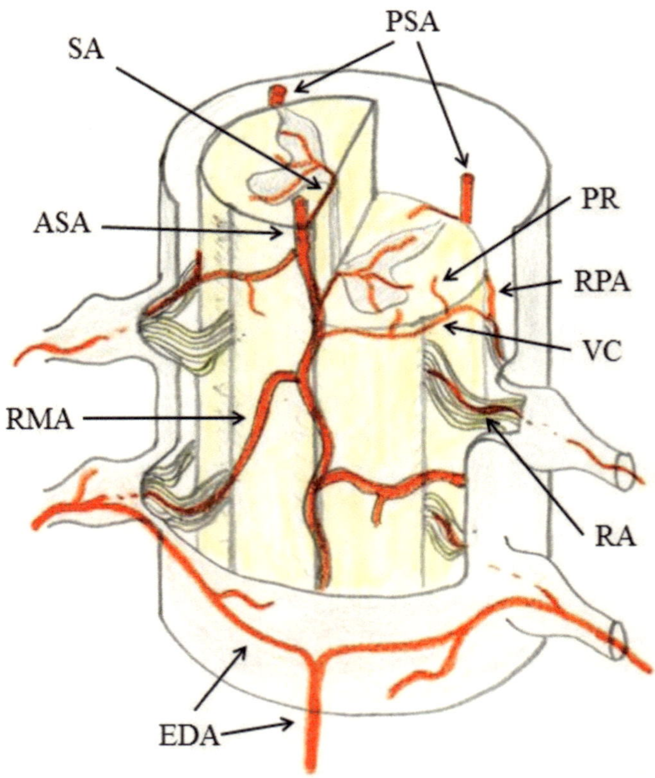

Figure 1. Arteries of the spinal cord. ASA: anterior spinal artery, PSA: posterior spinal artery, RMA: radiculomedullary artery, RPA: radiculopial artery, RA: radicular artery, SA: sulcal artery, VC: vasacorna, PR: perforating ramus, EDA: epidural anastomosis.

3. Classification of spinal AV shunts

3.1. Previous classifications

Many different classifications have been proposed for spinal AV shunts in terms of their location, vascular structure, and pathophysiology [16-23].

Rosenblum *et al.* classified spinal AV shunts into four types, on the basis of their angioarchitecture and clinical manifestations (Table 1) [16]. This simple classification is reasonable and has been widely used. However, it is hard to distinguish between type II (glomus-type malformations) and type III (juvenile-type malformations) in various preoperative examinations. The difficulty of treatment, prognosis, and onset pattern were not reflected in this classification.

Type I: Dural AV fistula
Type II: Glomus-type intradural AV malformation
Type III: Juvenile-type intradural AV malformation
Type IV: Intradural AV fistula
a : simple extramedullary fistulas fed by a single arterial branch
b : intermediate-sized fistulas with multiple, dilated arterial feeders
c : giant multipediculated fistulas

Table 1. Classification by Rosenblum *et al.*

Spetzler *et al.* advocated a classification system dependent on radiological and intraoperative findings, which closely reflects the difficulty of treatment (Table 2) [17, 18]. This classification, mainly intended as an aid to the open surgery, was noted for its anatomical detail of the shunts and a new categorization of "conus medullaris AV malformations." Unfortunately, different pathologies are ascribed to the same group in this classification, which can create confusion. For example, spinal dural AV fistulas and fistulous spinal cord AV malformations on the dorsal surface of the spinal cord belong to the same category (intradural dorsal AV fistulas).

AV fistulas	
	Extradural
	Intradural
	Ventral (small shunt, medium shunt, large shunt)
	Dorsal (single feeder, multiple feeders)
AV malformations	
	Extradural-intradural
	Intradural
	Intramedullary
	Compact
	Diffuse
	Conus medullaris
Neoplastic vascular lesions	
	Hemangioblastoma
	Cavernous malformation
Spinal aneurysms	

Table 2. Classification by Spetzler *et al.*

Rodesch *et al.* classified spinal AV shunts into the following three groups from genetic and hereditary points of view (Table 3) [19, 20]: (1) Genetic hereditary lesions that are caused by a genetic disorder affecting the vascular germinal cells. Spinal cord malformations associated with hereditary hemorrhagic telangiectasia (HHT) fall into this category. (2) Genetic nonhereditary lesions (such as somatic mutations) that share metameric links, including the Cobb syndrome, affecting the whole myelomere. Patients typically present with multiple shunts of the spinal cord, nerve root, bone, paraspinal muscle, subcutaneous tissue, and the skin. Klippel-Trenaunay and Parkes-Weber syndromes also belong to this group. (3) If there is no evidence of genetic disorder, a lesion is assumed to be a single lesion. It is likely that some of these isolated, apparently sporadic lesions may represent incomplete phenotypic expressions of an underlying, undiagnosed genetic or segmental syndrome. This classification reflects the important embryologic aspects of AV shunts; however, most cases (>80%) fall into the last group, which is not advantageous for treatment.

Genetic hereditary lesions : macrofistulae and hereditary hemorrhagic telangiectasia
Genetic nonhereditary lesions : all of which were multiple lesions with metameric or myelomeric associations
Single lesions : which could represent incomplete presentations of one of the above groups

Table 3. Classification of Rodesch *et al.*

Similar to pathology of the brain, spinal AV shunts can be differentiated into dural AV fistulas and spinal cord pial (intraparenchymal) AV malformations, depending on the shunt location and its related angioarchitecture [16, 24].

Spinal dural AV fistulas are fed by the radicular arteries and/or the surrounding vertebral branches, whereas spinal cord pial AV malformations are, similar to their cerebral counterparts, fed by the perimedullary and/or intrinsic arteries of the spinal cord. Spinal cord pial AV malformations may be either of the fistulous type, consisting of a direct connection between artery and vein, or of the nidus type, with an intervening network of vessels. Fistulas are further subdivided into micro- and macrofistulas. Nidi are further subdivided into glomus and juvenile types. Generally, dural AV fistulas are considered an acquired pathology, whereas pial AV malformations are presumed to be inborn vascular lesions.

The term "angioarchitecture" not only describes the morphology of the lesion at a given time, but also places the lesion in a temporal sequence. Most spinal AV shunts induce changes over time; marked venous ectasias may develop, and additional arterial feeders may be recruited. Venous thrombosis may induce spontaneous regression of the lesions. The type of shunt may remain fixed, but some fistulas may approach the nidus-type of malformation with time as a result of extensive pial reflux or intense intrinsic network congestion. The type of shunt implies the clinical presentation, treatment, and prognosis [20].

3.2. Spinal dural AV fistulas

Spinal dural AV fistulas account for 70% of all spinal AV shunts. Men are affected approximately five times more often than women. The disease usually becomes symptomatic in the elderly population. Most fistulas are located in the thoracolumbar region. Multiple fistulae in the same patient are exceedingly rare [25, 26].

Recently, both cranial and spinal dural AV fistulas have been categorized into ventral, dorsal, and lateral groups on the basis of the embryologic development of the venous drainage [27].

The ventral group consists of dural AV fistulas into those veins that normally drain the structures developed from the notochord (i.e., the vertebral body at the spinal level). These veins are known as the basivertebral venous plexus, which subsequently drains into the anterior internal vertebral venous plexus, located in the ventral epidural space of the spinal canal, which joins the basilar venous plexus and cavernous sinus. They may become symptomatic as a result of compression of the spinal cord or nerve roots by the enlarged epidural venous pouches. Because of the antireflux mechanism, these shunts do not induce the venous congestion of the spinal cord. There have been only a few case reports describing associated perimedullary reflux as a cause of congestive myelopathy. A hypothesis about a possible defect in the valve-like mechanism that normally impedes retrograde flow from the epidural plexus to perimedullary veins has been suggest to explain this finding.

The dorsal group of dural AV fistulas is related to veins that normally drain the spinous process and lamina at the spinal level. Although they are related to the major dural venous sinuses (superior sagittal sinus, torcular herophili, and transverse sinuses) at the cranial level, the corresponding veins at the spinal level are poorly developed and consist of a pair of longitudinal channels (i.e., the posterior internal venous plexus). Patients with dural AV fistulas within this space typically present with spontaneous epidural hematomas. These symptomatic lesions are extremely rare.

The most common "classic" type of spinal dural AV fistulas is categorized as the lateral group. This type represents >90% of all spinal dural AV fistulas that develop in the lateral epidural space at the junction of the veins that connect the spinal cord drainage to the epidural venous system. The fistula is located at the dura mater close to the spinal nerve root, where a radicular artery enters a radicular vein. Obstruction of its adjacent venous outlet, as a result of thrombosis or fibrosis related to aging, will lead to reflux into the perimedullary veins. Increase in spinal venous pressure diminishes the arteriovenous pressure gradient that leads to decreased drainage of normal spinal veins and venous congestion with intramedullary edema. This in turn leads to chronic hypoxia and progressive myelopathy. As a result, patients within this group present with aggressive clinical symptoms and at an older age. A strong male predominance is also observed, which is similar to that seen in the cranially located lateral AV fistulas, such as in the foramen magnum (medulla bridging vein) and tentorial (petrosal bridging vein) locations.

Symptoms of congestive myelopathy are unspecific. Usually, the deficits progress gradually; however, acute disease onset and progressive development interrupted by intermediate remissions is also possible. Mass effects and hemorrhagic changes are rare as presenting symptoms. Without therapy, the prognosis of this disease is grim, because it results in irreversible motor weakness, sensory disturbance, and bladder-bowel dysfunction [25, 26].

There are two options in the treatment of spinal dural AV fistulas; surgical occlusion of the intradural reflux vein, and endovascular therapy employing embolic material into the fistula. Surgery is a relatively simple and safe intervention, resulting in long-term shunt occlusion in

98% of cases [28]. In endovascular therapy, the embolic glue material must pass the fistula and occlude the proximal segment of the draining vein to prevent subsequent intradural collateral filling of the fistula. The success rates of endovascular therapy have been reported to vary between 25% and 75% [29-31]. Following complete occlusion of the fistula, the progression of the disease may cease; however, only two-third of all patients show regression of their motor weakness and only one-third show an improvement in sensory disturbances. Impotence and sphincter disturbances are seldom reversible [26].

3.3. Spinal cord pial AV malformations

Approximately 20%–30% of all spinal AV shunts are spinal cord pial AV malformations [16, 24, 32]. Similar to brain AV malformations, they are fed by arteries of the spinal cord and drained by spinal cord veins. These high-flow shunts might be intra- and/or perimedullary in location and can be differentiated into fistulous, glomus, and juvenile types, according to their shunt type and hemodynamic flow pattern. Fistulous and glomus types are often present within different compartments of the same AVM.

Fistulous AV malformations ("perimedullary AV fistulas") are direct AV shunts located superficially on the spinal cord and can possess intramedullary compartments. The shunt may be supplied by the anterior or posterior spinal artery, while the draining veins are the superficial perimedullary veins. This type can be subdivided into three types depending on the size of the feeding vessel, the volume of the shunt, and the drainage pattern [21]. Type I fistulas are small AV malformations; neither the feeding artery nor the draining vein is dilated, and the shunt volume is low. Type II fistulas are medium-sized AV malformations fed by one or two dilated arteries, whereas type III fistulas harbor multiple massively dilated arterial feeders and have a large shunt volume.

Glomus AV malformations have a nidus closely resembling that of a brain AV malformation and usually having an intramedullary location. The superficial nidus compartments may also reach the subarachnoid space. Because of the many anastomoses between the anterior and posterior arterial feeding systems of the spine, this type is typically fed by multiple arteries derived from both the anterior and the posterior systems. Drainage is into dilated vessels of the spinal cord.

Juvenile AV malformations are typically large with both fistulous and glomus compartments not only involving the spinal cord but also neighboring tissues such as the dura, vertebral body, and paravertebral muscle.

Venous congestion, hemorrhage, space-occupying effects and vascular steal have been attributed to the pathogenesis of spinal cord AV malformations. If the AV malformation does not present initially with an acute hemorrhage, symptoms are unspecific. The glomus type tends to become symptomatic in younger children and adolescents, whereas the fistulous type becomes symptomatic in young adults [16, 31].

The first attempt at treatment of spinal cord pial AV malformations tends to be an endovascular procedure, with the exception of most of type I fistulous AV malformations. Direct microsurgery should be conducted in type I fistulous malformations because the small caliber of the feeding artery prohibits placement of a catheter close to the fistula. Type II and III fistulous malformations have dilated feeding vessels enabling superselective catheterization close to the fistula and subsequent obliteration. In the glomus type, glue or particles can be employed to obliterate the nidus. In the juvenile type, only those parts of the malformation should be treated that are most likely to account for the symptoms [22-24].

4. Diagnostic imaging

When spinal lesions are suspected, MRI should constitute the first diagnostic modality.

In spinal dural AV fistulas, MRI demonstrates the combination of intramedullary signal alterations and perimedullary dilated vessels [25]. On T2-weighted images, the cord shows centromedullary hyperintensity over multiple segments. On T1-weighted images, the swollen cord is slightly hypointense and enlarged. Following contrast administration, diffuse intramedullary enhancement may be seen as a sign of chronic venous congestion with a breakdown of the blood–spinal cord barrier. In the further course of the disease, the spinal cord will be atrophic. The dilated and tortuous perimedullary vessels are mainly on the dorsal part of the cord and can be seen on the T2- weighted images as flow void signals. If they are small, however, they might be seen only after contrast enhancement. The coiled or serpentine vascular structures may be well delineated on heavily T2-weighted sequences. Shunts may occur anywhere from the level of the foramen magnum to the sacrum, and localization of these lesions may be difficult and challenging, especially in cases in which the edematous change of the cord occurs at a considerable distant from the shunt.

The typical appearance of spinal cord pial AV malformations is a conglomerate of dilated vessels with peri- and intramedullary locations that appear on T2-weighted images as flow void signals [32, 33]. Depending on their flow velocity and direction, these abnormal vessels are delineated as mixed hyper/hypointense tubular structures on T1-weighted images. Contrast enhancement may vary. Venous congestive edema may be present as an intramedullary hyperintensity on T2-weighted images with concomitant swelling of the cord. The image might become even more complicated if hematomyelia and subarachnoid hemorrhage are present; that might demonstrate varying signal intensities depending on the time course. MRI can identify the location of the nidus in relation to the spinal cord and dura. Especially in the small perimedullary fistulous type (type I), contrast media must be given to detect subtle venous dilatations.

Spinal contrast-enhanced dynamic MRA has contributed to shunt localization in some cases [34-37]. The technique of first-pass gadolinium-enhanced MRA can demonstrate early venous filling, which indicates the level of the shunt. Multidetector-row helical CT angiography with intravenous contrast injection (IV-CTA) can provide spinal vessel images showing the surrounding bony structure [38, 39]. These images allow a wide survey of possible shunts, but the spatial and temporal resolution is inadequate for planning the treatment strategy. Furthermore, cine review of the entire spine is not possible because of the limitations of acquisition time and the limited field of view (FOV).

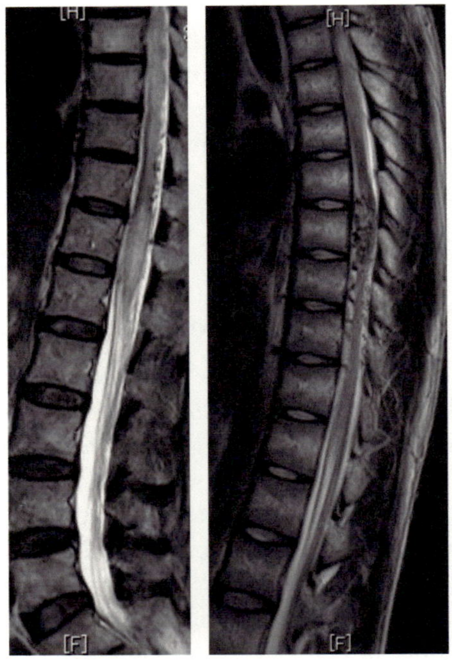

Figure 2. Sagittal sections of T2-weight MRI. Left: spinal dural AV fistula. Right: spinal cord AV malformation.

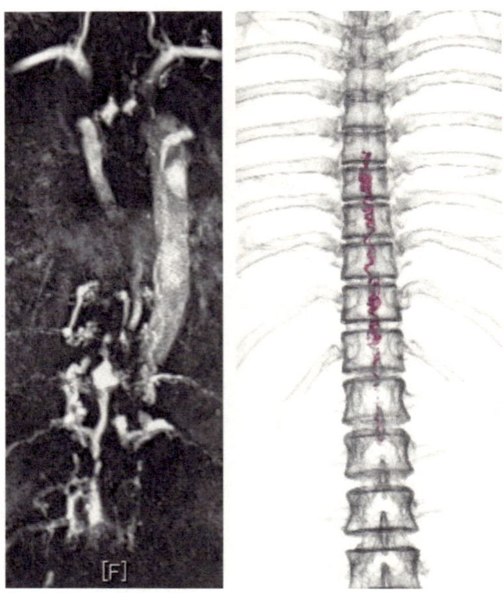

Figure 3. Less-invasive spinal vascular imagings. Left: Spinal contrast-enhanced dynamic MRA of fistulous-type spinal cord AV malformation (type III). Right: Multidetector-row helical CT angiography with intravenous contrast injection (IV-CTA) of fistulous-type spinal cord AV malformation (type II).

Although MRI, MRA and IV-CTA have the distinct advantage of less-invasive examination of the spinal cord and surrounding structures, their findings do not provide any hemodynamic information. Until date, selective spinal digital subtraction angiography (DSA) is the standard (and indispensable) for diagnosis, treatment, and follow-up examination of spinal vascular lesions [24, 37]. However, spinal DSA is an invasive procedure. Complete spinal DSA includes all vessels that may feed the spinal cord, i.e., all intercostal and lumbar arteries, the cervical feeders including both vertebral arteries, the thyrocervical trunk, the deep cervical artery, and the internal iliac arteries. Selective angiography of all segmental arteries can often be time-consuming, require multiple catheterizations, involve long radiation exposure times, and use large volumes of contrast agents. Furthermore, multiple catheterizations of small segmental arteries can lead to vessel injury and thromboembolism [40, 41].

5. Intra-arterial (intra-aortic) contrast injection CT angiography

Anatomical localization of the shunts is not only imperative for definitive therapy but can also complement spinal DSA, possibly leading to reduction in the number of selective catheterizations and fewer procedural complications. The radicular and spinal arteries are small vessels with a diameter of 0.5–1.5 mm and are surrounded by osseous structures. This anatomic feature decrease the contrast-to-noise ratio (CNR) in IV-CTA [42]. Although robust contrast enhancement is necessary for detection of small vessels, IV-CTA has limitations with respect to elevating vessel enhancement, because the contrast material is diluted in pulmonary circulation [43]. To delineate such minute vessels, a method that increases the bolus characteristic of contrast medium is preferable. To enhance the spatial resolution of spinal CTA, we tried multiphase intra-arterial (intra-aortic) contrast injection CT angiography (IA-CTA) in advance of spinal DSA. We found that IA-CTA could track the normal/abnormal spinal arteries to the aorta in detail. Multiphase dynamic imaging can discriminate the arterial component from the draining veins, which improves the precision of diagnosis.

A 4 (or 5) Fr Pigtail Catheter was advanced to the proximal portion of the descending aorta for thoracolumbar lesions or the proximal portion of the ascending aorta for cervicothoracic lesions. Patients were then transferred to the CT room, and 80 mL of iodinated contrast material (Iopamiron 300 mg I/ml; Nihon Schering K.K., Osaka, Japan) was injected via the catheter at a rate of 4 mL/s. The CT scan started 5 seconds after starting the injection and was consecutively repeated to obtain early- and late-phase images. Two datasets were reconstructed from the two consecutive scans. Image datasets were transferred to a workstation. An oblique coronal multiplanar reconstruction fitting the curvature of the spine was obtained. Exactly the same MPR sections were obtained from the second phase to distinguish the feeding arteries from the draining veins, which were in close proximity. Curved planar reformation (CPR) and three-dimensional volume rendering were applied to display an overview of the lesions. Detection of the arterial feeders confirmed the presence of a connecting vessel ascending from the intervertebral foramen to the lesions, and the absence of further enhancement in the second phase compared with the first phase. Continuity was confirmed by paging oblique coronal MPR or axial images. Spinal DSA with selective catheterization was subsequently performed with reference to the findings of IA-CTA.

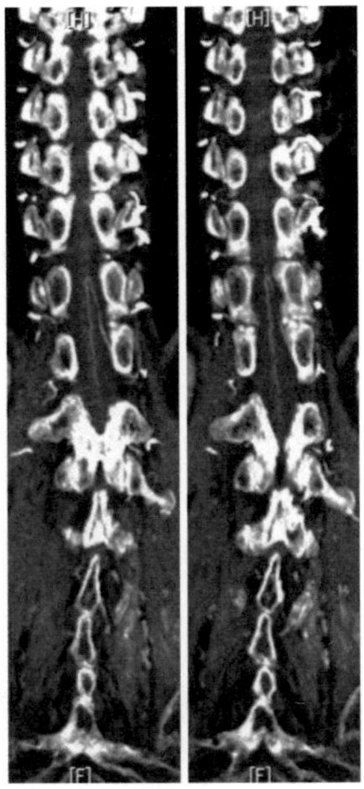

Figure 4. IA-CTA (arterial phase) demonstrating the radicular arteries and the artery of Adamkiewicz clearly.

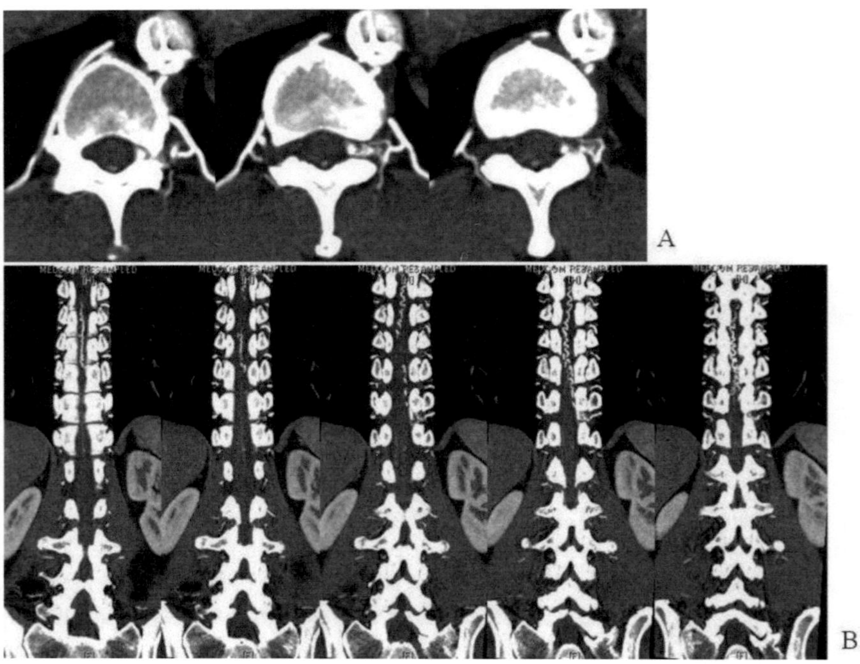

Figure 5. Spinal dural AV fistula with a feeder originated from the left T11 intercostal artery. A: serial axial sections of IA-CTA. B: serial coronal sections of IA-CTA.

http://dx.doi.org/10.5772/56367

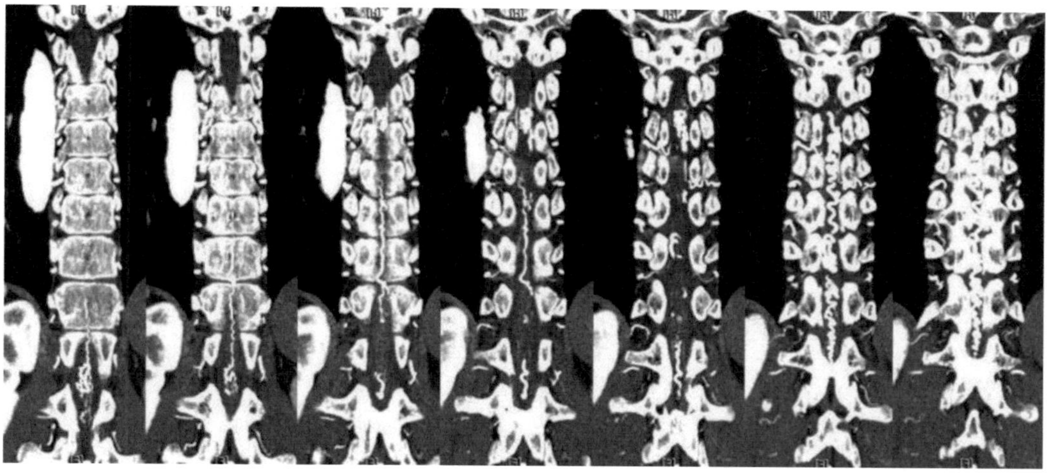

Figure 6. Serial coronal sections of IA-CTA demonstrating fistulous-type spinal cord AV malformation (type II), fed by rt. T9 and lt. T8 intercostal arteries.

6. Direct surgery under the guidance of intra-arterial injection indocyanine green (ICG) videoangiography

The goal of treatment for spinal AV shunts is the extirpation of shunt vessels without compromising the spinal cord circulation. In spinal cord pial AV malformations in particular, however, this is not feasible because of the complexity of the vasculature. For direct surgery of spinal cord AV shunts, various intraoperative diagnostic modalities have been used to assess the hemodynamics and to identify the shunting vessels, such as intraoperative spinal DSA, Doppler ultrasonography and videoangiography using indigo carmine and indocyanine green [44-50]. Intraoperative spinal DSA is a standard tool for demonstrating shunting flow and confirming extirpation [49]. However, its resolution is not adequate to assess the precise anatomy of the vasculature. Intra-arterial injection of indigo carmine via a catheter introduced for the spinal DSA has the advantage of visibility with conventional light optics; however, when compared with ICG fluorescence, the development and washout of the blue dye is less clear, and the time resolution and utility in discerning arterial or venous components is significantly limited [45]. Recent advances in microscope-integrated videoangiography using ICG have made it possible to visualize blood flow and hemodynamic changes in real time. A technique using intravenous injection of ICG has been used for cerebrovascular surgery, however, it is limited to detect the flow direction and velocity and to repeat the examination frequently [46-48]. To enhance the temporal and spatial resolution of this technique in spinal vascular surgery, we introduced intraarterial injection ICG videoangiography with selective catheterization [50].

After induction of general anesthesia, a 5-Fr long metallic introducer vessel sheath was inserted into the femoral artery in the operating room. After surgical exposure of the lesions, an

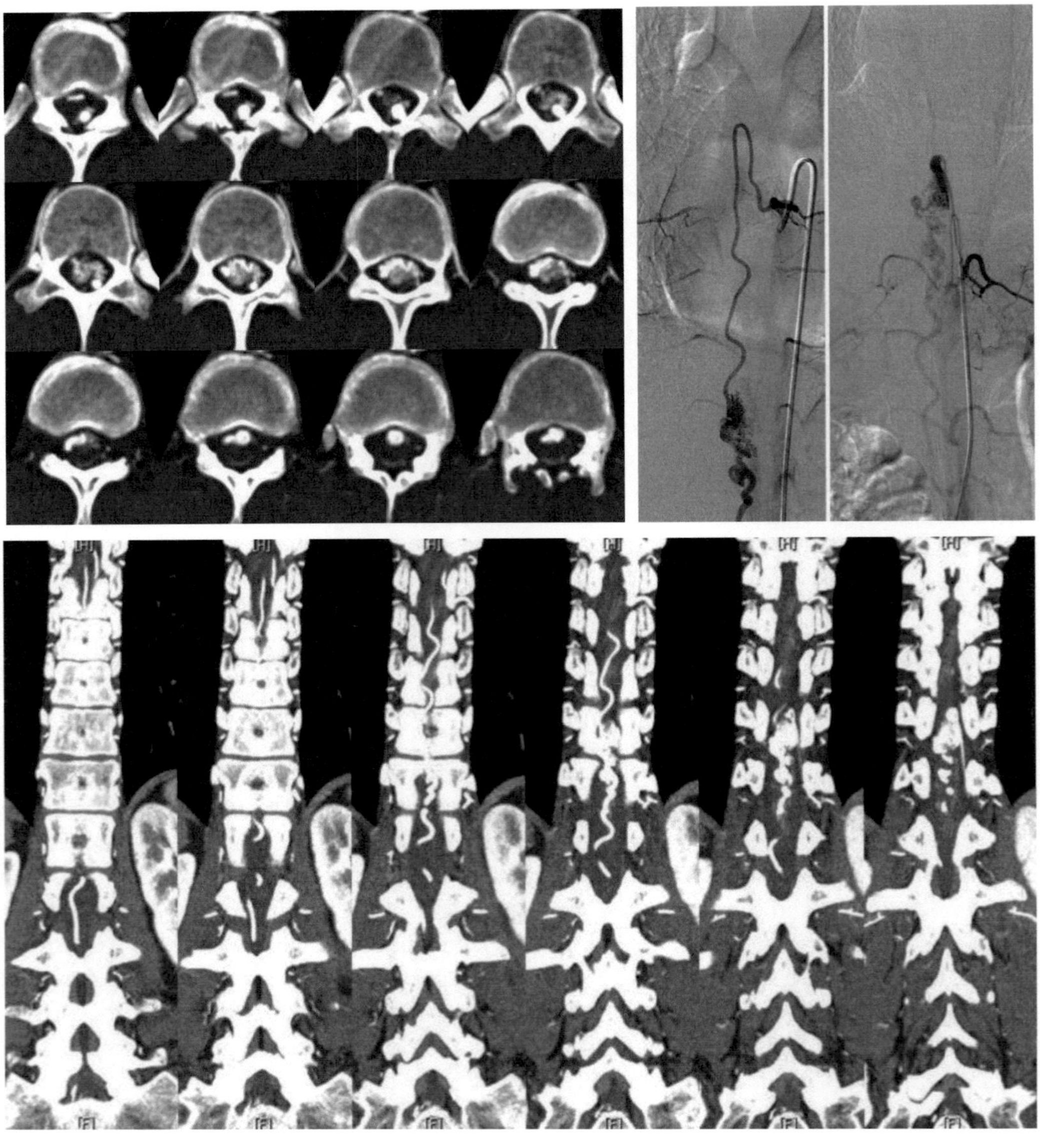

Figure 7. Glomus-type spinal cord AV pial malformation. Serial axial sections of IA-CTA showing the location of the intramedullary nidus and perimedullary varix. Coronal sections indicating 2 arterial feeders originated from the left T8 and T12 intercostal arteries, which was confirmed by spinal DSA.

angiographic catheter was placed into the proximal portion of the feeding artery for intraoperative DSA and ICG injection. When ICG solution (0.06 mg in 5 ml saline) was injected through the catheter, the feeders and then the drainers were illuminated with fluorescence and became clearly distinguishable using a fluorescence surgical microscope. Temporary occlusion applied close to the shunts led to immediate disappearance of the shunt flow. In addition to

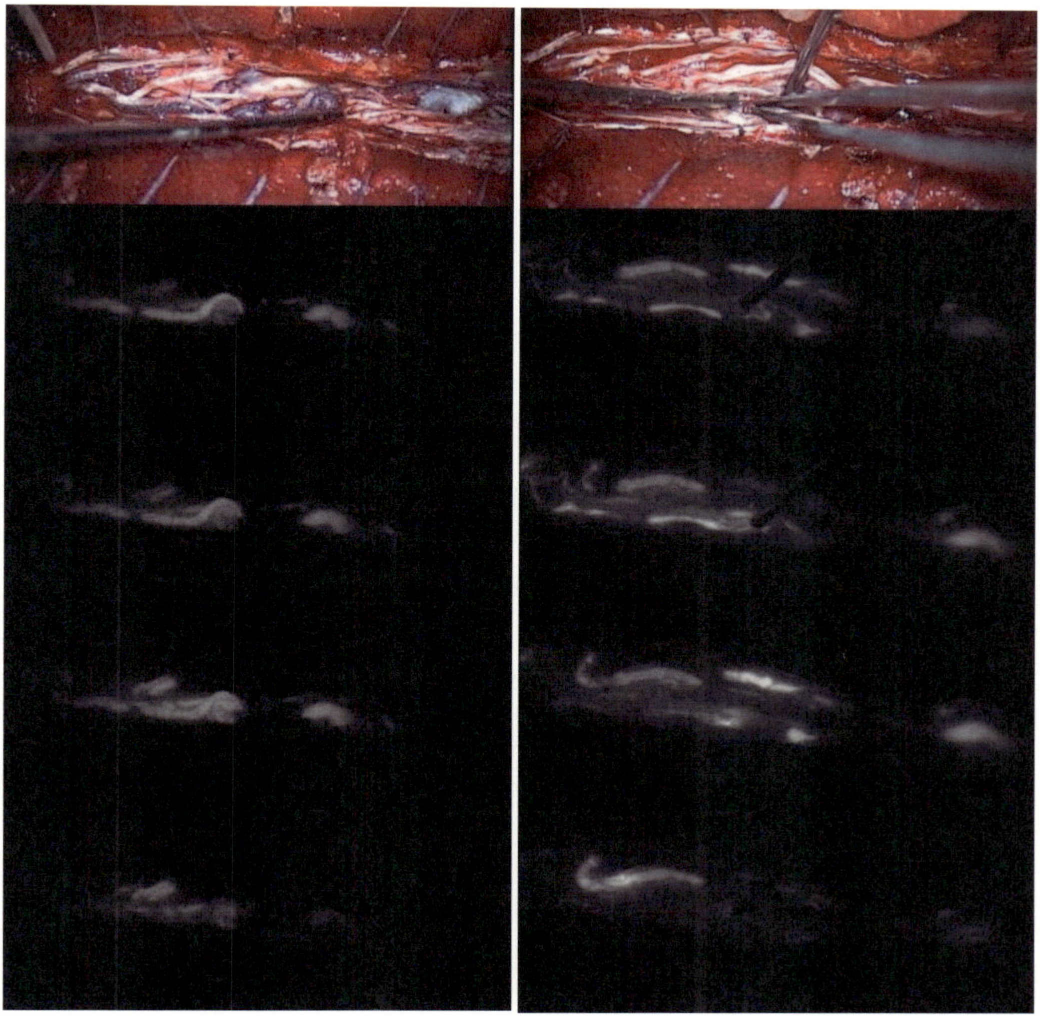

Figure 8. Intraoperative views of spinal cord AV malformation at the conus medullaris. Left: Indigo carmine videoangiography and serial photographs of IA-ICG videoangiography illuminating the feeders, shunts, and drainers in order. Right: IA-ICG videoangiography demonstrating the intraoperative flow alteration clearly.

fluorescence angiography, Doppler ultrasonography and intraoperative DSA were used to confirm extirpation of the AV shunts. Selective IA-ICG videoangiography also showed the patency of the normal anterior/posterior spinal artery, which could not be visualized by intraoperative DSA.

ICG videoangiography by intravenous bolus injection is performed with 10–25 mg ICG dissolved in saline. Once ICG is injected intravenously, the dye is diluted in the systemic circulation and carried to the tributary of observation via arterial flow. The background fluorescence remains for several minutes until the systemic concentration of ICG was decreased through hepatic excretion, which disturbed the detection of alterations in vessel flow. By using intra-arterial selective catheterization to the vicinity of the pathology, a much smaller dose of ICG can visualize the vessels without any background. Flow dynamics such as direction, velocity and alteration after temporary occlusion were well visualized. The resulting quick washout allows differentiation of the phase of the filling, thus identifying the feeder, the drainer, and the shunts in between. The small dose allows repetition of the examinations. The temporal resolution is far superior to that obtained by the intravenous injection technique. With test occlusion applied to one surface vessel to the other, and by observing alterations in the filling pattern in a real time, it becomes possible to identify the feeders and the drainers and thereby localize the embedded shunts. These are the great advantages of the intra-arterial injection over intravenous administration. The feasibility of multiple repeated injections helps in obtaining precise flow-dynamic information. When faced with complex spinal cord AV malformations, such repeated real-time information is indispensable for the localization and obliteration of the hidden shunts.

7. Conclusion

Despite the considerable advances that have been made in imaging and endovascular technology, spinal AV shunts continue to pose significant therapeutic challenges. Endovascular therapy and direct surgery with effective intraoperative diagnostic aids have a complementary role in the management, and understanding of the pathophysiology of these shunts and information about the detailed vasculature of the lesions is indispensable for achieving optimal results.

Author details

Shinji Yamamoto and Phyo Kim

Department of Neurologic Surgery, Dokkyo University, Tochigi, Japan

References

[1] Aminoff MJ, Barnard RO, Logue V. The pathophysiology of spinal vascular malformations. J Neurol Sci. 1974 Oct;23(2):255-63.

[2] Aminoff MJ, Logue V. Clinical features of spinal vascular malformations. Brain. 1974 Mar;97(1):197-210.

[3] Aminoff MJ, Logue V. The prognosis of patients with spinal vascular malformations. Brain. 1974 Mar;97(1):211-8.

[4] Detweiler PW, Porter RW, Spetzler RF. Spinal arteriovenous malformations. Neurosurg Clin N Am. 1999 Jan;10(1):89-100.

[5] Grote EH, Voigt K. Clinical syndromes, natural history, and pathophysiology of vascular lesions of the spinal cord. Neurosurg Clin N Am. 1999 Jan;10(1):17-45.

[6] Baker HL, Jr., Love JG, Layton DD, Jr. Angiographic and surgical aspects of spinal cord vascular anomalies. Radiology. 1967 Jun;88(6):1078-85.

[7] Cahan LD, Higashida RT, Halbach VV, Hieshima GB. Variants of radiculomeningeal vascular malformations of the spine. J Neurosurg. 1987 Mar;66(3):333-7.

[8] Di Chiro G, Doppman J, Ommaya AK. Selective arteriography of arteriovenous aneurysms of spinal cord. Radiology. 1967 Jun;88(6):1065-77.

[9] Djindjian M, Djindjian R, Rey A, Hurth M, Houdart R. Intradural extramedullary spinal arterio-venous malformations fed by the anterior spinal artery. Surg Neurol. 1977 Aug;8(2):85-93.

[10] Krayenbuhl H, Yasargil MG, McClintock HG. Treatment of spinal cord vascular malformations by surgical excision. J Neurosurg. 1969 Apr;30(4):427-35.

[11] Krings T. Vascular Malformations of the Spine and Spinal Cord : Anatomy, Classification, Treatment. Clin Neuroradiol. 2010 Feb 28. [Epub ahead of print]

[12] Lasjaunias PL, Berenstein A, terBrugge K. Surgical neuroangiography, vol 1. Clinical vascular anatomy and variations. Berlin: Springer, 2001. Apr;30(4):427-35.

[13] Zawilinski J, Litwin JA, Nowogrodzka-Zagorska M, Gorczyca J, Miodonski AJ. Vascular system of the human spinal cord in the prenatal period: a dye injection and corrosion casting study. Ann Anat. 2001 Jul;183(4):331-40.

[14] Tadie M, Hemet J, Freger P, Clavier E, Creissard P. Morphological and functional anatomy of spinal cord veins. J Neuroradiol. 1985;12(1):3-20.

[15] Krings T, Mull M, Bostroem A, Otto J, Hans FJ, Thron A. Spinal epidural arteriovenous fistula with perimedullary drainage. Case report and pathomechanical considerations. J Neurosurg Spine. 2006 Oct;5(4):353-8.

[16] Rosenblum B, Oldfield EH, Doppman JL, Di Chiro G. Spinal arteriovenous malformations: a comparison of dural arteriovenous fistulas and intradural AVM's in 81 patients. J Neurosurg. 1987 Dec;67(6):795-802.

[17] Spetzler RF, Detwiler PW, Riina HA, Porter RW. Modified classification of spinal cord vascular lesions. J Neurosurg. 2002 Mar;96(2 Suppl):145-56.

[18] Kim LJ, Spetzler RF. Classification and surgical management of spinal arteriovenous lesions: arteriovenous fistulae and arteriovenous malformations. Neurosurgery. 2006 Nov;59(5 Suppl 3):S195-201; discussion S3-13.

[19] Rodesch G, Hurth M, Alvarez H, Tadie M, Lasjaunias P. Classification of spinal cord arteriovenous shunts: proposal for a reappraisal--the Bicetre experience with 155 con-

secutive patients treated between 1981 and 1999. Neurosurgery. 2002 Aug;51(2): 374-9; discussion 9-80.

[20] Rodesch G, Hurth M, Alvarez H, Ducot B, Tadie M, Lasjaunias P. Angio-architecture of spinal cord arteriovenous shunts at presentation. Clinical correlations in adults and children. The Bicetre experience on 155 consecutive patients seen between 1981-1999. Acta Neurochirur. 2004 Mar;146(3):217-26; discussion 26-7.

[21] Mourier KL, Gobin YP, George B, Lot G, Merland JJ. Intradural perimedullary arteriovenous fistulae: results of surgical and endovascular treatment in a series of 35 cases. Neurosurgery. 1993 Jun;32(6):885-91; discussion 91.

[22] Patsalides A, Knopman J, Santillan A, Tsiouris AJ, Riina H, Gobin YP. Endovascular treatment of spinal arteriovenous lesions: beyond the dural fistula. Am J Neuroradiol. 2011 May;32(5):798-808.

[23] Zozulya YP, Slin'ko EI, Al Q, II. Spinal arteriovenous malformations: new classification and surgical treatment. Neurosurg focus. 2006;20(5):E7.

[24] da Costa L, Dehdashti AR, terBrugge KG. Spinal cord vascular shunts: spinal cord vascular malformations and dural arteriovenous fistulas. Neurosurg focus. 2009 Jan; 26(1):E6.

[25] Krings T, Geibprasert S. Spinal dural arteriovenous fistulas. Am J Neuroradiol. 2009 Apr;30(4):639-48.

[26] Fugate JE, Lanzino G, Rabinstein AA. Clinical presentation and prognostic factors of spinal dural arteriovenous fistulas: an overview. Neurosurg focus. 2012 May; 32(5):E17.

[27] Geibprasert S, Pereira V, Krings T, Jiarakongmun P, Toulgoat F, Pongpech S, et al. Dural arteriovenous shunts: a new classification of craniospinal epidural venous anatomical bases and clinical correlations. Stroke. 2008 Oct;39(10):2783-94.

[28] Steinmetz MP, Chow MM, Krishnaney AA, Andrews-Hinders D, Benzel EC, Masaryk TJ, et al. Outcome after the treatment of spinal dural arteriovenous fistulae: a contemporary single-institution series and meta-analysis. Neurosurgery. 2004 Jul;55(1): 77-87; discussion -8.

[29] Niimi Y, Berenstein A, Setton A, Neophytides A. Embolization of spinal dural arteriovenous fistulae: results and follow-up. Neurosurgery. 1997 Apr;40(4):675-82; discussion 82-3.

[30] Song JK, Vinuela F, Gobin YP, Duckwiler GR, Murayama Y, Kureshi I, et al. Surgical and endovascular treatment of spinal dural arteriovenous fistulas: long-term disability assessment and prognostic factors. J Neurosurg. 2001 Apr;94(2 Suppl):199-204.

[31] Van Dijk JM, terBrugge KG, Willinsky RA, Farb RI, Wallace MC. Multidisciplinary management of spinal dural arteriovenous fistulas: clinical presentation and long-term follow-up in 49 patients. Stroke. 2002 Jun;33(6):1578-83.

[32] Krings T, Mull M, Gilsbach JM, Thron A. Spinal vascular malformations. Eur Radiol. 2005 Feb;15(2):267-78.

[33] Doppman JL, Di Chiro G, Dwyer AJ, Frank JL, Oldfield EH. Magnetic resonance imaging of spinal arteriovenous malformations. J Neurosurg. 1987 Jun;66(6):830-4.

[34] Ali S, Cashen TA, Carroll TJ, McComb E, Muzaffar M, Shaibani A, et al. Time-resolved spinal MR angiography: initial clinical experience in the evaluation of spinal arteriovenous shunts. Am J Neuroradiol. 2007 Oct;28(9):1806-10.

[35] Farb RI, Kim JK, Willinsky RA, Montanera WJ, terBrugge K, Derbyshire JA, et al. Spinal dural arteriovenous fistula localization with a technique of first-pass gadolinium-enhanced MR angiography: initial experience. Radiology. 2002 Mar;222(3):843-50.

[36] Mull M, Nijenhuis RJ, Backes WH, Krings T, Wilmink JT, Thron A. Value and limitations of contrast-enhanced MR angiography in spinal arteriovenous malformations and dural arteriovenous fistulas. Am J Neuroradiol. 2007 Aug;28(7):1249-58.

[37] Zampakis P, Santosh C, Taylor W, Teasdale E. The role of non-invasive computed tomography in patients with suspected dural fistulas with spinal drainage. Neurosurgery. 2006 Apr;58(4):686-94; discussion -94.

[38] Lai PH, Pan HB, Yang CF, Yeh LR, Hsu SS, Lee KW, et al. Multi-detector row computed tomography angiography in diagnosing spinal dural arteriovenous fistula: initial experience. Stroke. 2005 Jul;36(7):1562-4.

[39] Si-jia G, Meng-wei Z, Xi-ping L, Yu-shen Z, Jing-hong L, Zhong-hui W, et al. The clinical application studies of CT spinal angiography with 64-detector row spiral CT in diagnosing spinal vascular malformations. Eur J Radiol. 2009 Jul;71(1):22-8.

[40] Forbes G, Nichols DA, Jack CR, Jr., Ilstrup DM, Kispert DB, Piepgras DG, et al. Complications of spinal cord arteriography: prospective assessment of risk for diagnostic procedures. Radiology. 1988 Nov;169(2):479-84.

[41] Kieffer E, Fukui S, Chiras J, Koskas F, Bahnini A, Cormier E. Spinal cord arteriography: a safe adjunct before descending thoracic or thoracoabdominal aortic aneurysmectomy. J Vasc Surg. 2002 Feb;35(2):262-8.

[42] Yoshioka K, Niinuma H, Ehara S, Nakajima T, Nakamura M, Kawazoe K. MR angiography and CT angiography of the artery of Adamkiewicz: state of the art. Radiographics. 2006 Oct;26 Suppl 1:S63-73.

[43] Nakayama Y, Awai K, Yanaga Y, Nakaura T, Funama Y, Hirai T, et al. Optimal contrast medium injection protocols for the depiction of the Adamkiewicz artery using 64-detector CT angiography. Clinical radiology. 2008 Aug;63(8):880-7.

[44] Iacopino DG, Giusa M, Conti A, Cardali S, Tomasello F. Intraoperative microvascular Doppler monitoring of blood flow within a spinal dural arteriovenous fistula: a precious surgical tool. Case report. Neurosurg focus. 2001;10(2):ECP1.

[45] Tani S, Ikeuchi S, Hata Y, Abe T. Vascular orientation by intra-arterial dye injection during spinal arteriovenous malformation surgery. Neurosurgery. 2001 Jan;48(1): 240-2.

[46] Colby GP, Coon AL, Sciubba DM, Bydon A, Gailloud P, Tamargo RJ. Intraoperative indocyanine green angiography for obliteration of a spinal dural arteriovenous fistula. J Neurosurg Spine. 2009 Dec;11(6):705-9.

[47] Hanel RA, Nakaji P, Spetzler RF. Use of microscope-integrated near-infrared indocyanine green videoangiography in the surgical treatment of spinal dural arteriovenous fistulae. Neurosurgery. May;66(5):978-84; discussion 84-5.

[48] Murakami T, Koyanagi I, Kaneko T, Iihoshi S, Houkin K. Intraoperative indocyanine green videoangiography for spinal vascular lesions: case report. Neurosurgery. 2011 Mar;68(1 Suppl Operative):241-5; discussion 5.

[49] Schievink WI, Vishteh AG, McDougall CG, Spetzler RF. Intraoperative spinal angiography. J Neurosurg. 1999 Jan;90(1 Suppl):48-51.

[50] Yamamoto S, Kim P, Kurokawa R, Itoki K, Kawamoto S. Selective intraarterial injection of ICG for fluorescence angiography as a guide to extirpate perimedullary arteriovenous fistulas. Acta Neurochir. 2012 Mar;154(3):457-63.

Chapter 6

Spinal Arteriovenous Fistulas

Mohammad R. Rasouli, Vafa Rahimi-Movaghar and
Alexander R. Vaccaro

Additional information is available at the end of the chapter

http://dx.doi.org/10.5772/56729

1. Introduction

Spinal cord vascular lesions can be broadly classified into one of the 3 following groups: neoplasm (hemangioblastomas and cavernous malformations), aneurysms, and arteriovenous malformations (AVM).[1],[2] Spinal AVMs account for 1% to 2% of vascular neurologic pathologies and 3%-12% of space-occupying pathologies of the spinal cord.[3]

Several classifications have been proposed for spinal AVMs.[2],[4]-[6] They can be divided into intramedullary AVMs and arteriovenous fistulas (AVFs). Based on anatomical characteristics, spinal AVFs are classified as extradural AVFs and intradural lesions, including spinal dural AVFs (SDAVFs) and perimedullary spinal AVFs (PMAVFs).[7],[8] Rangel-Castilla et al. classified extradural AVFs as type A or type B based on the availability of intradural venous drainage. In Type A spinal extradural AVFs, there is intradural venous drainage and arterio-venous shunting develops in the epidural space. Type B can be further classified as B1 and B2, both of which are limited to the epidural space without any intradural draining veins. The only difference between these two types is the presence or absence of compression on the spinal cord and nerve roots.[9] There is a paucity of literature about spinal AVFs and due to the very small incidence of these lesion, almost all available studies are small cases series. However, spinal AVFs can manifest with severe neurologic symptoms, leading to permanent neurologic deficit. Therefore, in this chapter we aim to review the available literature about spinal AVFs.

2. Literature search

A literature search of Medline through PubMed was performed using following search terms: ("Arteriovenous Malformations"[Mesh] OR "Arteriovenous Fistula"[Mesh]) AND "Spinal

Cord." Then we limited our search to English-language articles and studies on human subjects. We expanded our literature search using the "related citation" option in PubMed. We also searched Google Scholar using the following keywords: spinal, arteriovenous fistula, extra-dural arteriovenous fistula, spinal dural arteriovenous fistula, and perimedullary spinal arteriovenous fistula. We also manually searched the reference lists of important papers to identify those that we missed during our primary electronic search. Data on epidemiology, classification, etiology, clinical manifestations, diagnosis, management, prognostic factors, and outcome of SDAVFs were extracted from selected articles.

3. SDAVFs

Although SDAVFs are rare, they are the most common spinal vascular malformation and are responsible for 70% of spinal cord arteriovenous shunts,[10] with an annual incidence of 5-10 cases per million.[11] It has been suggested that SDAVFs are acquired lesions, though their exact etiology remains unknown. SDAVFs are seen more frequently in elderly males and tend to affect the thoracolumbar segment more frequently than other spinal segments.[10]

SDAVFs are low-flow lesions and cause venous hypertension and chronic spinal cord hypoxia. Patients present with progressive myelopathy. Paraparesis is often the initial presentation, which is followed by root and/or back pain, sensory impairment, and sphincter dysfunction. [7]Due to non-specific presentations, SDAVFs are often diagnosed late. The mean time interval between onset of symptoms and diagnosis of SDAVF has been reported as high as 22.9 months (range 12 to 44 months).[12]-[14] Some authors suggest that there is a correlation between time until diagnosis of SDAVF and severity of symptoms.[5],[15] As mentioned earlier, the majority of authors consider SDAVFs to be acquired lesions and that they should be differentiated from congenital intradural PMAVFs.[16]

Digital subtraction angiography is the gold standard for diagnosis of spinal vascular malformations, including SDAVF[17]; however, magnetic resonance imaging (MRI) has been suggested as an accurate and reliable tool for diagnosis of SDAVF.[7] Intramedullary high-intensity changes on T2-weighted MRI are seen when SDAVF is present.[18] After treatment of SDAVF, intramedullary high-intensity changes start to reduce in the majority of cases between 1 and 4 months after treatment and these changes disappear in most cases between 2 weeks and 23 months after treatment. Although there is a possible correlation between the severity of these changes and preoperative neurologic deficits, there is not necessarily an association between reduction of intramedullary changes and clinical improvement.[18] One of the radiologic findings correlating with severity of functional status of patients with SDAVF is craniocaudal extension of the enlarged intrathecal draining veins.[19] For diagnosis of residual or recurrent flow in peri- or intramedullary vessels after treatment of SDAVFs, magnetic resonance angiography (MRA) may be more sensitive than MRI.[20]

SDAVFs can be treated surgically, endovascularly embolized, or a combination of surgery and endovascular techniques may be used.[21],[22] Traditionally, surgery is considered the treatment of choice for SDAVFs. If the lesion can be localized using imaging studies preoperatively, surgery can be performed with a low complication rate.[22] In comparison, endovascular approaches are less invasive. However, surgery has an advantage over endovascular techniques when there are multiple SDAVFs because surgery provides direct visibility of all feeding vessels. Since the first case of surgical treatment of SDAVF in 1916,[23] advances in treatment have led to simplified techniques and good outcomes. Nowadays, the typical surgical approach consists of a posterior approach with a laminectomy or hemilaminotomy. The dura is opened, the arterialized vein is identified, and either cauterization or microscissor interruption of the SDAVF is performed.[13],[24],[25] Compared to clipping the draining vein alone, excision or coagulation of the nidus and disconnection of the draining vein may be associated with more favorable long-term results.[26] Complications following surgery are rare; however, instability after laminectomy and pseudomeningocele are two potential complications that can be minimized by limited facet removal (<50%) and meticulous closure of the dura, muscle, and skin.[24]

Endovascular techniques are less invasive and preserve spinal cord tissue and its function; in some cases, access to the feeding vessels of SDAVFs is not possible endovascularly.[22] The first case of SDAVF embolization using metal pellets was described in 1968 by Doppman et al. [27] Since then, new agents including polyvinyl alcohol (PVA), isobutyl-2-cyanoacrylate (IBCA), and N-butyl cyanoacrylate (NBCA) have been introduced and used for endovascular embolization of various vascular lesions including SDAVF.[13] Although the rate of recanalization following use of PVA was high (up to 93%),[28] the success rate of SDAVF embolization increased to 70%-90% using NCBA.[13] Ethylene vinyl alcohol (Onyx, EV3) liquid embolic system has also been used for embolization of SDAVFs. Onyx was approved by the Food and Drug Administration to be used for embolization of intracranial AVMs but has been used for treatment of spinal AVFs in recent years.[29]-[31] Onyx, which is a nonadhesive liquid agent, carries the advantages of lower likelihood of adhesion of the catheter to the vessels, which facilitates the injection of a larger amount of the agent.[30] In a small series of 3 SDAVFs, Nogueira et al. reported successful management of SDAVF without evidence of residual or recurrent AVF confirmed clinically and radiologically (MRI and MRA) during follow up of more than 7 months.[29] In another small series of 6 patients with SDAVF, Carlson et al. reported complete occlusion of AVF in 5 of the patients during 2 to 4 months of follow up using the Onyx embolization system.[32] It seems that in the future, Onyx will be the preferred embolization method for management of SDAVFs.

In a 2004 meta-analysis, Steinmetz et al. suggested that for treatment of SDAVF, surgery might be superior to embolization. Surgery is usually successful and recurrence and complications are rare. The authors also suggested that endovascular intervention might be a reasonable initial option; however, this technique is associated with a relatively high rate of recurrence. [24] Nowadays, in spite of significant improvements in endovascular embolization and the introduction of new embolization agents, surgery still seems to be the treatment of choice.[13] After treatment, the majority of patients experience improvement; however, symptoms may remain unchanged or deterioration might occur in a few cases.[24],[33]Overall, if timely treatment occurs, patient outcomes for motor abilities and gait disability scores will be particularly good.[34] However, if urinary dysfunction occurs, it less likely responds to treatment.[35] It seems that time from onset of symptoms to treatment is the largest determinant of outcome in patients with SDAVF.

4. PMAVFs

In 1977, Djindjian and colleagues described PMAVFs for the first time. They described PMAVF as abnormal direct connections between the anterior spinal artery and/or posterior spinal artery and the medullary veins without any intervening nidus.[36] PMAVF is located on the pial surface of the spinal cord. Later, Heros et al. considered PMAVFs to be type IV spinal vascular malformations.[37] PMAVFs can be classified into type I, type II, or type III according to the size of the fistula, the number of feeding arteries, and the severity of venous hypertension.[6],[38]-[40]

Type I is a small and single AVF which is fed by the terminal segment of a thin anterior spinal artery. The anatomic location of the AVF is against the anterior surface of the conus medullaris or the filum terminale. Draining perimedullary veins are slightly dilated. Type I AVFs are hemodynamically similar to SDAVFs.

Type II is an intermediate-sized AVF and is fed by multiple arteries. The anatomic location of the AVF is against the conus medullaris. The shunt may be found more frequently in a posterolateral position and less frequently in the anterior position. In the posterolateral position, the feeding artery originates from ipsilateral posterior spinal artery. In anteriorly-located AVFs, the feeding artery originates from the anterior spinal artery. The AVF drains directly to a dilated and tortuous venous system containing a relatively high flow of arterialized blood. However, venous drainage in type II AVFs is slow.

Type III AVFs are large and single and located at the cervical or thoracic spinal cord. The AVF is fed by multiple arteries originating from the anterior and posterior spinal arteries. High-flow AVF drains to a very dilated and tortuous venous system.

The etiology of PMAVF is not clear. Although it is believed these lesions are congenital,[16] few cases of traumatic PMAVF have been reported in the literature.[39],[41] PMAVF is usually diagnosed between the third and sixth decades of life and are very rare, particularly in children.[42]The exact prevalence of PMAVFs is unknown but it is estimated that they constitute 4%-40% of spinal AVMs.[43],[44] Although the thoracolumbar spinal cord is the most common site of PMAVFs, these lesions can be seen at cervical and thoracic levels as well.[32]

PMAVFs are high-flow lesions leading to venous hypertension.[7] PMAVFs manifest with progressive myelopathy in the majority of patients and can result in complete transverse myelopathy if treatment does not occur.[44]Subarachnoid hemorrhage has also been reported in PMAVF cases.[39],[45] Due to non-specific presentation, the time from onset of symptoms to diagnosis may vary from 2 to 25 years.[46] Angiography is still the gold standard for diagnosis of PMAVF and its benefits include possible simultaneous treatment. However, angiography is invasive and time-consuming, and is only available in specialized centers.

Recent studies indicate that MRI has high sensitivity for diagnosis of spinal AVFs.[7] It is recommended that MRI be ordered as the initial imaging study, followed by MRA if necessary.

PMAVFs can be treated surgically, with endovascularly embolized, or combination of techniques can be performed.[47]-[50] Early diagnosis and treatment may be associated with better results and may prevent irreversible spinal cord injury. Removal of shunt vessels while the spinal cord perfusion is preserved is the purpose of surgery; however, sometimes complex vasculature of the shunt and risk of spinal cord perfusion impairment make surgery complicated. Therefore, various intraoperative diagnostic tools should be used to appropriately identify shunt vessels to avoid damaging spinal cord perfusion. Spinal cord angiography, Doppler ultrasound, and videoangiography using indigo carmine and indocyanine green are some of these modalities.[51]-[53]

Due to the paucity of literature on PMAVF, which results from the very low incidence and prevalence of these lesions, it is not possible to standardize surgical approaches for these lesions; therefore, a variety of surgical approaches have been used for management of them.[45],[54]-[56] For treatment of giant PMAVFs, a combination of surgery and endovascular embolization is recommended.[57],[58] Embolization of PMAVF can be performed using glue, coils, and balloons.[47],[50],[57] Overall, treatment of PMAVFs is more difficult than treatment of SDAVFs.[38] Because the majority of PMAVFs are high-flow shunts, endovascular embolization should be considered as the initial therapeutic modality in pediatric patients.[47] In summary, surgery is successful in the treatment of PMAVFs, even in cases with involvement of the anterior spinal artery. In high-flow PMAVFs, endovascular embolization is an appropriate adjunct to surgery.[59]

5. Extradural AVFs

Extradural AVFs are the least frequent type of spinal AVFs. In spinal extradural AVFs, a direct connection exists between the artery or arteries and the extradural venous plexus, which is not available in normal individuals. This abnormal connection is located within the spinal canal and/or intervertebral foramen. Extradural AVFs can cause venous hypertension, mass effect, and vascular steal leading to myelopathy.[8]

Type A extradural spinal AVFs usually manifest as congestive myelopathy or cauda equina syndrome based on the location of the AVF; however, type B1 extradural spinal AVFs present with spinal cord or nerve root compression. Type B2 extradural AVFs are asymptomatic.[30]MRI findings in Type A spinal extradural AVFs are spinal cord edema and perimedullary flow voids. On T2-weighted images, spinal cord edema (hyperintensity) is seen over multiple segments with a hypointense rim, most likely indicating deoxygenated blood.[8] In contrast, type B2 spinal extradural AVFs are difficult to diagnose with MRI and spinal angiography is the imaging modality of choice for diagnosis of these lesions.

Treatment consists of complete obliteration of the extradural AVF by either embolization or surgical excision.[8] It has been reported that after partial obliteration spinal extradural AVFs will recruit new blood supplies and make treatment more difficult. For management of Type A spinal extradural AVF it is not mandatory to occlude the intradural draining vein. However, it is necessary to inject embolic material into the entire malformation to achieve complete obliteration.[30]

Improvement of endovascular techniques and agents that are using for embolization of lesions may yield better results in the treatment of extradural AVFs. Recently, Rangel-Castilla used Onyx for the embolization of 7 extradural AVFs. Four patients had excellent recovery at 6-24 months and 3 patients with type A extradural AVF experienced good motor recovery without improvement of bladder/bowel problem.[9]

Author details

Mohammad R. Rasouli[1], Vafa Rahimi-Movaghar[2,3] and Alexander R. Vaccaro[1,4]

1 Rothman Institute of Orthopaedics, Thomas Jefferson University, Philadelphia, PA, USA

2 Sina Trauma and Surgery Research Center, Tehran University of Medical Sciences, Tehran, Iran

3 Department of Neurosurgery, Shariati Hospital, Tehran University of Medical Sciences, Tehran, Iran

4 Departments of Orthopaedic Surgery and Neurological Surgery, Thomas Jefferson University, Philadelphia, PA, USA

References

[1] Muralidharan R, Saladino A, Lanzino G, Atkinson JL, Rabinstein AA. The clinical and radiological presentation of spinal dural arteriovenous fistula. Spine (Phila Pa 1976). 2011;36:E1641-7.

[2] Spetzler RF, Detwiler PW, Riina HA, Porter RW. Modified classification of spinal cord vascular lesions. J Neurosurg. 2002;96:145-56.

[3] Matushita H, Caldas JG, Texeira MJ. Perimedullary arteriovenous fistulas in children: report on six cases. Childs Nerv Syst. 2012;28:253-64.

[4] Oldfield EH, Doppman JL. Spinal arteriovenous malformations. Clin Neurosurg. 1988;34:161-83.

[5] Westphal M, Koch C. Management of spinal dural arteriovenous fistulae using an interdisciplinary neuroradiological/neurosurgical approach: experience with 47 cases. Neurosurgery. 1999;45:451-7.

[6] Anson J, Spetzler RF: Classification of spinal arteriovenous malformations and implications of treatment. BNI Q. 1992; 8:2–8.

[7] Toossi S, Josephson SA, Hetts SW, Chin CT, Kralik S, Jun P, Douglas VC. Utility of MRI in spinal arteriovenous fistula. Neurology. 2012;79:25-30.

[8] Takai K, Taniguchi M. Comparative analysis of spinal extradural arteriovenous fistulas with or without intradural venous drainage: a systematic literature review. Neurosurg Focus. 2012;32:E8.

[9] Rangel-Castilla L, Holman PJ, Krishna C, Trask TW, Klucznik RP, Diaz OM. Spinal extradural arteriovenous fistulas: a clinical and radiological description of different types and their novel treatment with Onyx. J Neurosurg Spine. 2011;15:541-9.

[10] Krings T, Mull M, Gilsbach JM, Thron A. Spinal vascular malformations. Eur Radiol. 2005;15:267-78.

[11] Koch C. Spinal dural arteriovenous fistula. Curr Opin Neurol. 2006;19:69-75.

[12] Jellema K, Tijssen CC, van Gijn J. Spinal dural arteriovenous fistulas: a congestive myelopathy that initially mimics a peripheral nerve disorder. Brain. 2006;129:3150-64.

[13] Sivakumar W, Zada G, Yashar P, Giannotta SL, Teitelbaum G, Larsen DW. Endovascular management of spinal dural arteriovenous fistulas. A review. Neurosurg Focus. 2009;26:E15.

[14] Narvid J, Hetts SW, Larsen D, Neuhaus J, Singh TP, McSwain H, Lawton MT, Dowd CF, Higashida RT, Halbach VV. Spinal dural arteriovenous fistulae: clinical features and long-term results. Neurosurgery. 2008;62:159-66.

[15] Eskandar EN, Borges LF, Budzik RF Jr, Putman CM, Ogilvy CS. Spinal dural arteriovenous fistulas: experience with endovascular and surgical therapy. J Neurosurg. 2002 Mar;96:162-7.

[16] Sasaki O, Yajima N, Ichikawa A, Yamashita S, Nakamura K. Deterioration after surgical treatment of spinal dural arteriovenous fistula associated with spinal perimedullary fistula. Neurol Med Chir (Tokyo). 2012;52:516-20.

[17] Takai K, Kin T, Oyama H, Iijima A, Shojima M, Nishido H, Saito N. The use of 3D computer graphics in the diagnosis and treatment of spinal vascular malformations. J Neurosurg Spine. 2011;15:654-9.

[18] Horikoshi T, Hida K, Iwasaki Y, Abe H, Akino M. Chronological changes in MRI findings of spinal dural arteriovenous fistula. Surg Neurol. 2000;53:243-9.

[19] Hetts SW, Moftakhar P, English JD, Dowd CF, Higashida RT, Lawton MT, Douglas VC, Halbach VV. Spinal dural arteriovenous fistulas and intrathecal venous drainage: correlation between digital subtraction angiography, magnetic resonance imaging, and clinical findings. J Neurosurg Spine. 2012;16:433-40.

[20] Mascalchi M, Ferrito G, Quilici N, Mangiafico S, Cosottini M, Cellerini M, Politi LS, Guerrini L, Bartolozzi C, Villari N. Spinal vascular malformations: MR angiography after treatment. Radiology. 2001;219:346-53.

[21] Afshar JK, Doppman JL, Oldfield EH. Surgical interruption of intradural draining vein as curative treatment of spinal dural arteriovenous fistulas. J Neurosurg. 1995;82:196-200.

[22] Heldner MR, Arnold M, Nedeltchev K, Gralla J, Beck J, Fischer U. Vascular diseases of the spinal cord: a review. Curr Treat Options Neurol. 2012;14:509-20.

[23] Elsberg CA: Diagnosis and Treatment of Surgical Diseases of the Spinal Cord and Its Membranes. London, W.B. Saunders Co., 1916, pp 94–204.

[24] Steinmetz MP, Chow MM, Krishnaney AA, Andrews-Hinders D, Benzel EC, Masaryk TJ, Mayberg MR, Rasmussen PA. Outcome after the treatment of spinal dural arteriovenous fistulae: a contemporary single-institution series and meta-analysis. Neurosurgery. 2004;55:77-87.

[25] Desai A, Bekelis K, Erkmen K. Minimally invasive tubular retractor system for adequate exposure during surgical obliteration of spinaldural arteriovenous fistulas with the aid of indocyanine green intraoperative angiography. J Neurosurg Spine. 2012;17:160-3.

[26] Tacconi L, Lopez Izquierdo BC, Symon L. Outcome and prognostic factors in the surgical treatment of spinal dural arteriovenous fistulas. A long-term study. Br J Neurosurg. 1997;11:298-305.

[27] Doppman JL, Di Chiro G, Ommaya A. Obliteration of spinal-cord arteriovenous malformation by percutaneous embolisation. Lancet. 1968;1:477.

[28] Morgan MK, Marsh WR. Management of spinal dural arteriovenous malformations. J Neurosurg. 1989;70:832-6.

[29] Nogueira RG, Dabus G, Rabinov JD, Ogilvy CS, Hirsch JA, Pryor JC. Onyx embolization for the treatment of spinal dural arteriovenous fistulae: initial experience with long-term follow-up. Technical case report. Neurosurgery. 2009;64:E197-8.

[30] Rangel-Castilla L, Holman PJ, Krishna C, Trask TW, Klucznik RP, Diaz OM. Spinal extradural arteriovenous fistulas: a clinical and radiological description of different types and their novel treatment with Onyx. J Neurosurg Spine. 2011;15:541-9.

[31] Spiotta AM, Hughes G, Masaryk TJ, Hui FK. Balloon-augmented Onyx embolization of a dural arteriovenous fistula arising from the neuromeningeal trunk of the ascending pharyngeal artery: technical report. J Neurointerv Surg. 2011;3:300-3.

[32] Carlson AP, Taylor CL, Yonas H. Treatment of dural arteriovenous fistula using ethylene vinyl alcohol (onyx) arterial embolization as the primary modality: short-term results. J Neurosurg. 2007;107:1120-5.

[33] Schick U, Hassler W. Treatment and outcome of spinal dural arteriovenous fistulas. Eur Spine J. 2003;12:350-5.

[34] Rubin MN, Rabinstein AA. Vascular diseases of the spinal cord. Neurol Clin. 2013;31:153-81.

[35] Song JK, Vinuela F, Gobin YP, Duckwiler GR, Murayama Y, Kureshi I, Frazee JG, Martin NA. Surgical and endovascular treatment of spinal dural arteriovenous fistulas: long-term disability assessment and prognostic factors. J Neurosurg. 2001;94:199-204.

[36] Djindjian M, Djindjian R, Rey A, Hurth M, Houdart R. Intradural extramedullary spinal arterio-venous malformations fed by the anterior spinal artery. Surg Neurol. 1977;8:85-93.

[37] Heros RC, Debrun GM, Ojemann RG, Lasjaunias PL, Naessens PJ. Direct spinal arteriovenous fistula: a new type of spinal AVM. Case report. J Neurosurg. 1986;64:134-9.

[38] Merland JJ, Riche MC, Chiras J. Les fistules artérioveineuses intracanalaires extramédullaires à drainage veineux médullaire. J Neuroradiol. 1980; 7:271–320.

[39] Gueguen B, Merland JJ, Riche MC, Rey A. Vascular malformations of the spinal cord: intrathecal perimedullary arteriovenous fistulas fed by medullary arteries. Neurology. 1987;37:969–79.

[40] Mourier KL, Gobin YP, George B, Lot G, Merland JJ. Intradural perimedullary arteriovenous fistulae: results of surgical and endovascular treatment in a series of 35 cases. Neurosurgery. 1993;32:885-91.

[41] Meng X, Zhang H, Chen Y, Ling F. Traumatic spinal perimedullary arteriovenous fistula: a case report. Acta Neurochir (Wien). 2010;152:1407-10.

[42] Meng X, Zhang H, Wang Y, Ye M, He C, Du J, Ling F. Perimedullary arteriovenous fistulas in pediatric patients: clinical, angiographical, and therapeutic experiences in a series of 19 cases. Childs Nerv Syst. 2010;26:889-96.

[43] Matushita H, Caldas JG, Texeira MJ. Perimedullary arteriovenous fistulas in children: report on six cases. Childs Nerv Syst. 2012;28:253-64.

[44] Cho KT, Lee DY, Chung CK, Han MH, Kim HJ. Treatment of spinal cord perimedullary arteriovenous fistula: embolization versus surgery. Neurosurgery. 2005;56:232-41.

[45] Barrow DL, Colohan AR, Dawson R. Intradural perimedullary arteriovenous fistulas (type IV spinal cord arteriovenous malformations). J Neurosurg. 1994;81:221-9.

[46] Tomlinson FH, Rüfenacht DA, Sundt TM Jr, Nichols DA, Fode NC. Arteriovenous fistulas of the brain and the spinal cord. J Neurosurg. 1993;79:16-27.

[47] Lv X, Li Y, Yang X, Jiang C, Wu Z. Endovascular embolization for symptomatic perimedullary AVF and intramedullary AVM: a series and a literature review. Neuroradiology. 2012;54:349-59

[48] Mourier KL, Gobin YP, George B, Lot G, Merland JJ. Intradural perimedullary arteriovenous fistulae: results of surgical and endovascular treatment in a series of 35 cases. Neurosurgery. 1993;32:885-91.

[49] Pasqualetto L, Papa R, Isalberti M, Nuzzi NP, Branca V. The endovascular treatment of a spinal perimedullary arteriovenous fistula with coils: a case report. J Neurointerv Surg. 2011;3:88-91.

[50] Oran I, Parildar M, Derbent A. Treatment of slow-flow (type I) perimedullary spinal arteriovenous fistulas with special reference to embolization. AJNR Am J Neuroradiol. 2005;26:2582-6.

[51] Yamamoto S, Kim P, Kurokawa R, Itoki K, Kawamoto S. Selective intraarterial injection of ICG for fluorescence angiography as a guide to extirpate perimedullary arteriovenous fistulas. Acta Neurochir (Wien). 2012;154:457-63.

[52] Murakami T, Koyanagi I, Kaneko T, Iihoshi S, Houkin K. Intraoperative indocyanine green videoangiography for spinal vascular lesions: case report. Neurosurgery. 2011;68:241-5.

[53] Miyoshi Y, Yasuhara T, Nishida A, Tokunaga K, Sugiu K, Date I. Effectiveness of intraoperative near-infrared indocyanine green videoangiography in a case with recurrent spinal perimedullary arteriovenous fistula. Clin Neurol Neurosurg. 2011;113:239-42.

[54] Anderer EG, Kang MM, Moshel YA, Frempong-Boadu A. Successful management of an anterior thoracic Type IV spinal arteriovenous malformation with two associated aneurysms utilizing vertebrectomy. Technical note. J Neurosurg Spine. 2008;9:67-70.

[55] Martin NA, Khanna RK, Batzdorf U. Posterolateral cervical or thoracic approach with spinal cord rotation for vascular malformations or tumors of the ventrolateral spinal cord. J Neurosurg. 1995;83:254-61.

[56] Giese A, Winkler PA, Schichor C, Kantelhardt SR, Boeckh-Behrens T, Tonn JC, Rohde V. A transmedullary approach to occlusion of a ventral perimedullary arteriovenous fistula of the thoracic spinal cord. Neurosurgery. 2010;66:611-5.

[57] Casasco A, Guimaraens L, Senturk C, Cotroneo E, Gigli R, Theron J. Endovascular treatment of cervical giant perimedullary arteriovenous fistulas. Neurosurgery. 2012;70:141-9.

[58] Nagashima C, Miyoshi A, Nagashima R, Ogawa M, Enomoto K, Watabe T. Spinal giant intradural perimedullary arteriovenous fistula: clinical and neuroradiological study in one case with review of literature. Surg Neurol. 1996;45:524-31.

[59] Hida K, Iwasaki Y, Goto K, Miyasaka K, Abe H. Results of the surgical treatment of perimedullary arteriovenous fistulas with special reference to embolization. J Neurosurg. 1999;90:198-205.

Section 3

Systemic Arteriovenous Fistula

Chapter 7

Pulmonary and Other Non-Neurological Vascular Malformations: Diagnosis and Endovascular Treatment

Yasutaka Baba, Sadao Hayashi and
Masayuki Nakajo

Additional information is available at the end of the chapter

http://dx.doi.org/10.5772/56730

1. Introduction

Since the International Society for the Study of Vascular Anomalies (ISSVA) was founded in 1992, the confused classification of vascular anomalies has improved and classified into 2 major categories; vascular tumors and vascular malformations and arteriovenous malformation (AVM) or arteriovenous fistula (AVF) belong to vascular malformations [1]. Although there has been a definite differentiation of pathological and clinical findings between vascular tumors and vascular malformations [1], new findings of vascular malformations have trickled in by some recent molecular biological study of vascular malformation [2-6]. There appears no clear difference in definition between AVM and AVF at this moment. Therefore we used AVM or AVF interchangeably according to the involved organs and previous papers.

We present our experiences in diagnosis and endovascular treatment of non-neurological vascular malformations. First of all, we address diagnosis and endovascular treatment of pulmonary AVMs. The symptoms of pulmonary AVMs include hypoxia, hemo-sputum, hyper-coagulated state, and paradoxical embolism. In addition, exciting new knowledge of pulmonary AVMs, including hereditary factors and cytokines such as vascular endothelial growth factor (VGEF) releasing phenomenon within the venous sac, are now highlighted. Endovascular treatment and long term follow-up results of pulmonary AVMs are also discussed. About vascular malformations involving other organs, we will present and illustrate a wide spectrum of vascular malformations involving neck, extremity, liver, common bile duct, pancreas, kidney, intestine, pelvic and uterine.

2. Chest

2.1. Diagnosis and endovascular treatment of Pulmonary AVMs (PAVMs)

PAVMs are caused by abnormal communications between pulmonary arteries and pulmonary veins without the capillary beds and are most commonly congenital in nature. PAVMs are usually classified into the simple type with one feeding segmental artery and the complex type with 2 or more feeding segmental arteries. Definite diagnosis of PAVMs is made by contrast enhanced computed tomography and pulmonary angiography [7-9].

The right-to-left shunt causes the symptoms of PAVMs and results in hypoxia, dyspnea, cyanosis, and polycythemia when the shunt is developed. Besides this, lack of filter function due to absence of capillary beds induces the symptoms of paradoxical embolism and may results in brain abscess (10) or infarction. Although recently, small PAVMs are discovered on multi-detector row computed tomography (MDCT), the feeding pulmonary artery 3 mm or greater in diameter is generally indicated for treatment of PAVMs in order to block the nidus (sac) of PAVMs [9.11].

Embolotherapy has been the treatment option for PAVMs because it is minimally invasive, easy to perform and achieves a high success rate [7,8]. Microcoils have been used to treat PAVMs, but vascular plugs may be next generation devices to treat PAVMs [12]. However, incomplete occlusion of the sac or recanalization of an embolized feeding artery during a long-term follow-up could be seen in clinical setting. Remy-Jardin et al [7] reported that the overall treatment success rate was 75 % at long term follow- ups (2-21 years) and repeated embolotherapy was required for recanalized PAVM and occurred in 19 % patients. Meanwhile, Pollak et al [8] reported that problems related with embolized PAVMs occurred in 23 % of treated patients at several interval follow-up points (over 3-7 years) and symptomatic events related to recanalization included respiratory symptoms, cerebral ischemia, brain abscess, hemoptysis and seizure. Like Remy-Jardin et al.[7], Pollak et al [8] emphasized that early recognition of the recanalized sac on follow-up imaging modality (computed tomography) and repeated embolotherapy are necessary to prevent recurrent symptoms related with PAVMs. In our experience, the overall treatment success rate was 70 % at long term follow-up series (from 1989 to 2009) and the major cause of failed cases hinges on recanalized emolized arteries, in which repeated embolotherapy was required. However, symptoms related with recanalized PAVMs were not recognized in our series.

2.2. Sac Embolization is adequate strategy for treatment of PAVMs

We define here reperfusion as sac blood flow irrespective of the inflow route and recanalization as sac blood flow from the previously or successfully embolized arterial portion, respectively. Our colleagues [13] have reported a high rate (57 %) of reperfusion of PAVMs with steel coils and documented that the bronchial artery is one of the routes for reperfusion after embolotherapy for PAVMs. Therefore, we intend to embolize the sac itself with microcoils when the sac is 30 mm or less in diameter to prevent reperfusion in our institute. In the comparative study between the feeding artery embolization and sac embolization groups, the former showed a significant higher reperfusion rate at long term follow-ups (soon published). Reperfusion mainly depended on the type and number of used coils.

2.3. The causes of reperfusion of embolized PAVMs (Fig. 1)

Mechanisms underlying reperfusion of the embolized PAVMs were summarized by Pollak et al. [8] as: i) recanalization of the embolized vessel; ii) growth of a missed or previously small accessory artery; iii) bronchial and other systemic artery collateral flow into the pulmonary artery beyond the level of the embolization (creating a left-to-left shunt); and iv) pulmonary artery-to-pulmonary artery collateral flow about the occlusion. Reperfusion may occur individually or in combination of the aforementioned mechanisms. Mechanism iv, has been observed only in young children and presumably results from the ability for continued lung growth [8].

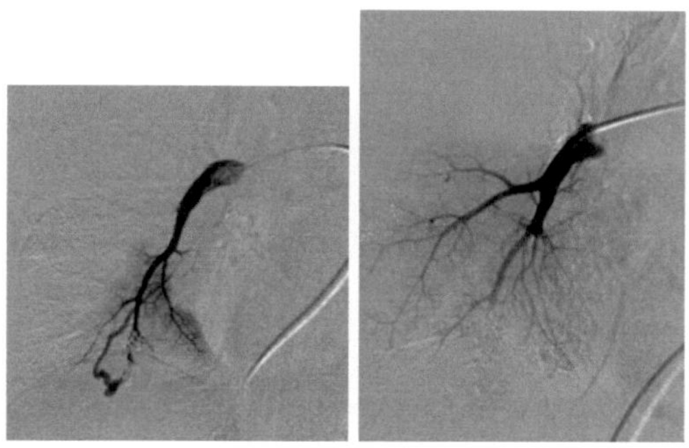

(a) (b)

Figure 1. Pulmonary AVM. (a) Right middle branch of pulmonary arteriogram shows recanalized nidus through the previous embolized feeding vessel with microcoils. (b) Right middle branch of pulmonary arteriogram shows complete embolized nidus after additional coil embolization.

2.4. Some cytokines are released via a sac?

Dupuis-Girod et al [6] have reported that bevacizumab has an effect on reducing the symptoms relating with high cardiac output or PAVMs regression in patients with PAVMs in hereditary hemorrhagic telangiectasia (HHT) that exhibits AVMs in several different organs. Some cytokines like VGEF and TGF beta may have relationship with development of pulmonary AVMs [2-6] and anti VGEF agents have a potential to regression of PAVMs [2]. However, Giordano et al mentioned that VGEF and TGF beta are not useful for diagnosing HHT [3].

2.5. Systemic circulation to thoracic AVMs (Fig.2)

Another specific type of thoracic AVMs is mediastinal AVM, which is difficult to manage the symptoms relating with high flow shunting, for example, hemoptysis and hemothorax [14]. Unlike PAVMs, the shunt blood flow is derived from systemic arterial blood flow and untreated various systemic arterial branches could develop even if embolotherapy is attempted. Therefore it is very hard to block the arterial blood inflow to the nidus, resulting in recurrent symptoms related with thoracic AVMs.

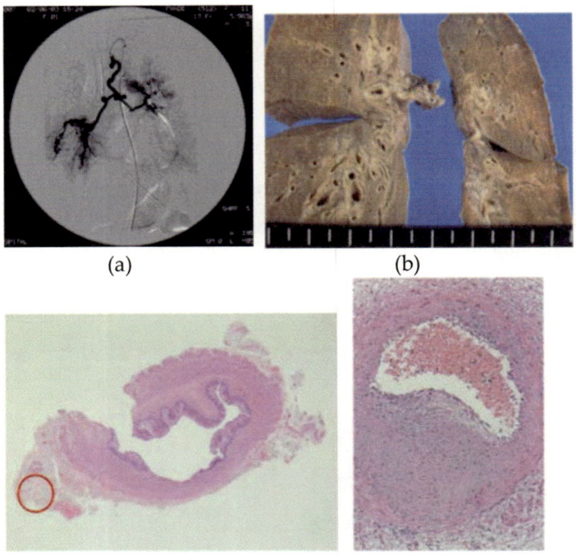

(a) (b) (c) (d)

Figure 2. Mediastinal AVMs.(a) Bronchial arteriogram shows neovascularization and patchy staining at bilateral lung hilum. There are many systemic arterial supplies to these mediastinal lesions (not shown). (b) Gross speciemen of the resected lungs show the hypertrophied bronchial walls and the hilums. (c) Microscopic speciemen of the resected esophagus shows neovascularization around the esophagus (red circle). (d) Microscopic speciemen in which red circle denotes reveals the proliferation of the vascular wall.

3. Other non-neurological AVFs

3.1. Neck AVMs (Fig.3)

Unlike other peripheral vascular AVMs, it is difficult to manage neck AVMs and control the symptoms. Particularly embolotherapy is difficult to perform because of high risk of cerebrovascular events after treatment and fortified vascular supply to the nidus, resulting in recurrent AVMs. Ordinal embolotherapy with gelatin, coils, and n-butyl cyanoacrylate (NBCA) could not become a breakthrough treatment option for head and neck AVMs. A recent clinical study showed that ethanol sclerotherapy is promising for treating head and neck AVMs [15]. Ethanol is a toxic substance that destroys the endothelial wall permanently and results in thrombus formation [16]. However, it needs to pay attention to blood flow speeds via the nidus because absolute ethanol has a risk of lethal direct tissue injury including pulmonary artery collapse [16]. Therefore, remission of blood flow via the nidus by an appropriate method (for instance, using balloon catheter, coils, or other liquid agents) is essential to exploit absolute ethanol.

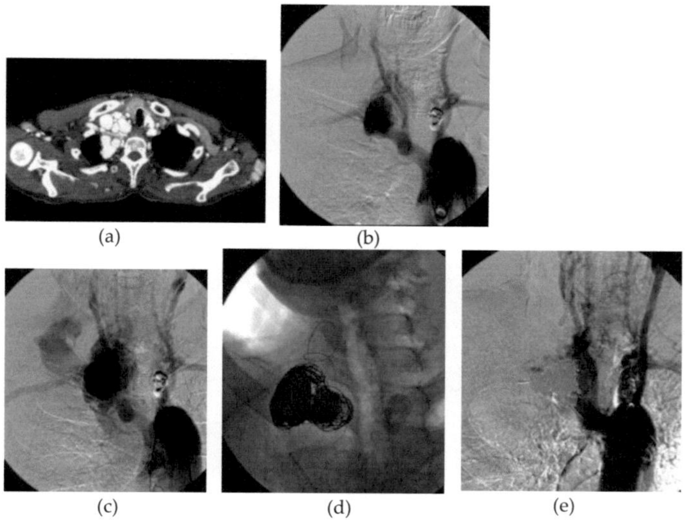

Figure 3. Neck AVMs. (a) Contrast enhanced computed tomography (CT) shows that torturous and dilated vessels at the right neck. (b) Aortogram shows neovascularization and dilated vessels around the right neck. (c) Aortogram also shows that early visualization of the dilated and torturous veins around the right neck. (d) Coil embolization via both arterial and venous sides was performed repeatedly. (e) After coil embolization, despite of incomplete embolization, aortogram shows the diminish blood flow via the nidus.

3.2. Liver AVFs: HCCs/ HHT (Fig.4)

In patients with HHT, liver is frequently involved and they show a wide spectrum of clinical manifestations. In patients with HHT, traces of elements that pass through hepatic AVMs, could affect the extrapyramidal movement via depositing manganese in the globus pallidus [17]. On the contrary, hepatocellular carcinomas (HCC) easily invades hepatic venous structures according to its progression, result in hepatic arteriovenous fistulas. In patients with AV fistulas due to HCC, it is difficult to treat them by embolotherapy because fistula channels are derived from tumor vasculatures. We experienced a case of HCC whose AV fistula was successfully treated by absolute ethanol [18].

3.3. Common bile ducts AVFs: Hereditary Hemorrhagic Telangiectasia (HHT) (Fig.5)

HHT involves rarely the common bile duct. Hemobilia may occur because AVMs may protrude from the common bile duct wall. We experienced a patient with HHT who had a small AVM of the common bile duct causing intractable hemobilia [19].

Later, intractable hemobilia ceased by superselective coil embolization (Fig.5) and have not recurred. Other clinical findings associated with HHT, for instance, intractable epistaxis, telangiectasis of the lip, tongue, and oral cavity might be key to reach the etiology of hemobilia. Otherwise, it is difficult to recognize the imaging findings associated with HHT except selective angiography.

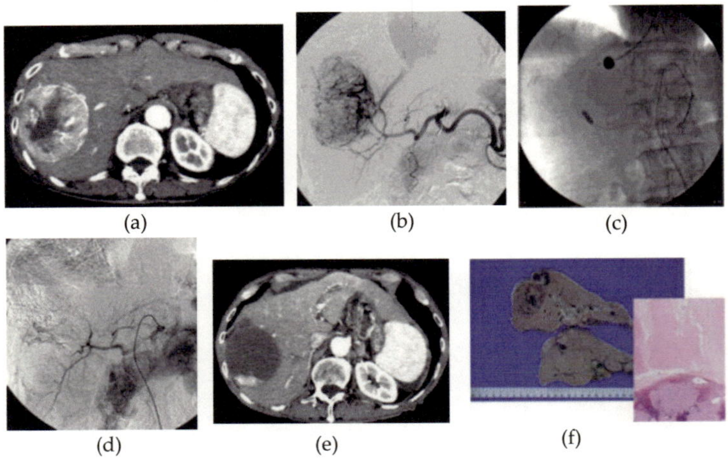

Figure 4. Hepatocellular carcinoma with arteriovenous shunting. (All figures are cited under permission from publishing company: reference 18) (a) Contrast enhanced CT shows the hypervascular tumor in the right liver lobe. (b) Celiac arteriogram shows not only the hypervascular liver tumor but also early visualization of the right hepatic vein. (c) We attempted to embolize intratumoral shunting by way of combined balloon inflation via both hepatic arterial and venous sides. Under this condition, the intratumoral shunting can be embolized with absolute etanol. (d) After embolization with absolute ethanol, celiac arteriogram shows vanishing of intratumoral shunting and hypervascular liver tumor. (e) After these procedures, on contrast enhanced CT, the vast majority of hypervascualr tumor shows necrosis. (f) On macroscopic (left) and microscopic (right) specimens of the resected liver, the major part of the liver tumor shows necrosis. Reproduced from reference [18] with the permission of the publisher.

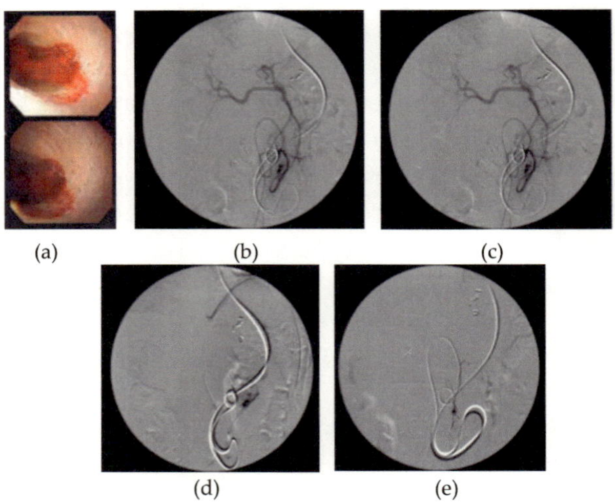

Figure 5. AVMs of common bile duct in a patient with hereditary hemorrhagic telangiectasis. (All figures are cited under permission from publishing company: reference 19) (a) Bile duct endoscopy shows bleeding in the bile duct lumen. (b) Inferior pancreaticoduodenal arteriogram shows patchy stain in the lower bile duct. (c) Selective arteriogram via the branch of pancreaticoduodenal arcade shows the staining in the lower bile duct. (d) After coil embolization of bleeding sites, the staining in the lower bile duct disappeared on amgiogram. Reproduced from reference [19] with the permission of the publisher.

http://dx.doi.org/10.5772/56730

3.4. Pancreatic AVFs: Post transplantation and Metastasis from Renal Cell Carcinoma (RCC)

Apart from the case with HHT, postoperative pancreatic transplantation is the major cause of pancreas AVFs [20]. Another cause of pancreatic AVFs is metastatic pancreatic cancer from renal cell carcinoma. In both entities of pancreatic AVF, it could be difficult to manage the portal hypertension symptoms associated with inflowing systemic blood pressure to the portal system. Barth et al. [20] reported that elegant embolization via both transarterial and transvenous accesses for the pancreatic AVF case.

3.5. Intestinal AVMs

In the patients with obscure origin of gastrointestinal bleeding (GIB), small intestinal AVM is one of the sources that cause intractable GIB. Coil embolization of angiodysplasia have been reported, however, embolothearpy may not always successful to cease GIB and surgical intervention sometimes may be necessary [21-23].

When operation is performed in a patient with intestinal AVMs, placing coils might be help to recognize the location of intestinal AVMs.

3.6. Colonic AVMs (Fig.6)

Colonic AVM is rare and could induce portal hypertension and coil embolization may be feasible to treat it [24]. We experience a patient with rectal AVFs whose major part was thrombosed and calcified, but intractable rectal bleeding continued. Curative operation was performed later, the sysmptom associated with rectal AVF was resolved.

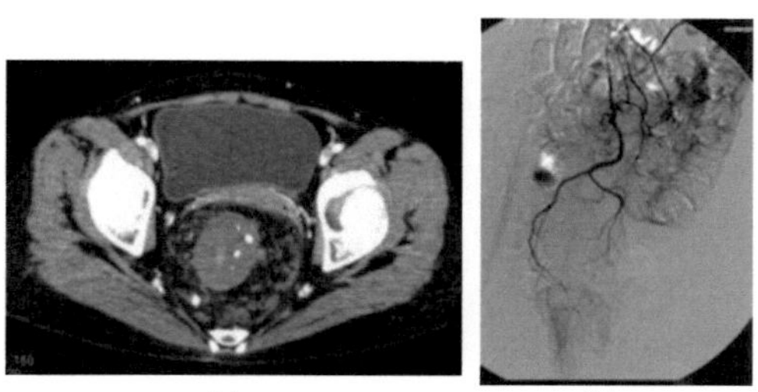

(a) (b)

Figure 6. Rectal AVMs. (a) Contrast enhanced computed tomography (CT) shows no enhanced, thickening and calcified mass of the rectum, which was surrounded by pararectal venous varices. (b) Superior rectal arteriogram shows minor tumor staining without early venous drainage. Therefore, thrombotic change was suspected in the major part of arteriovenous malformation.

3.7. Renal AVMs/AVFs (Fig.7,8)

Renal AVF is a frequent disease but may be misdiagnosed unless classical findings of renal AVFs are depicted on ultrasonography (US) or contrast enhanced CT. We misdiagnosed renal AVF in a patient in whom contrast CT depicted aneurysmal dilatation at the level of renal hilum [25]. In renal AVFs/AVMs, embolotherapy could be a major option to treat and occlude the fistula or nidus.

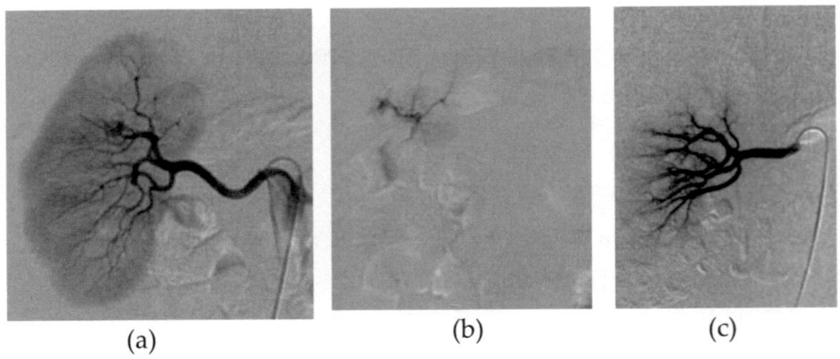

Figure 7. Renal AVM; (a) Right renal arteriogram shows staining of the upper pole of the kidney.(b) Early venous drainage is evident on super-selective arteriogram of the upper pole of the renal artery. (c)After embolization of the renal AVM with absolute ethanol, it disappeared.

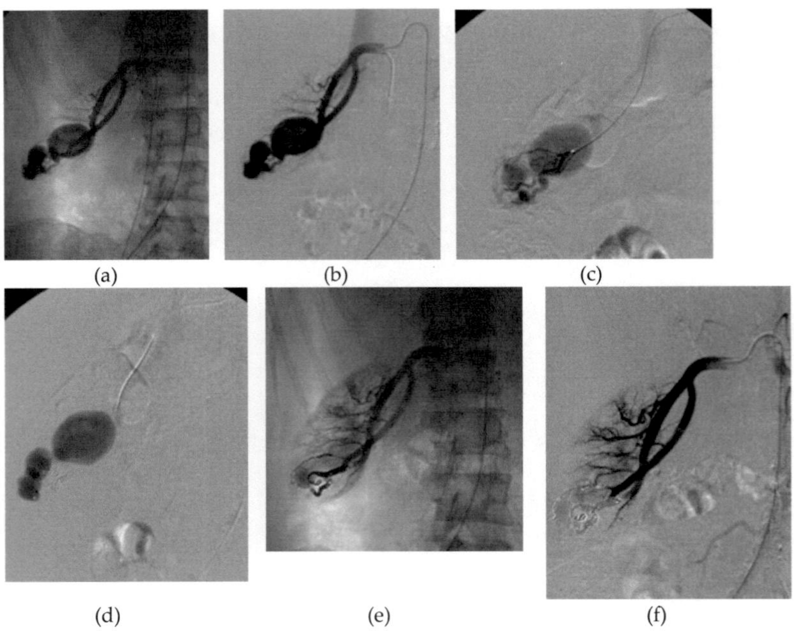

Figure 8. Renal AVF with venous aneurismal dilatation.(a)(b) Right renal arteriogram shows the hypertrophied renal artery and aneurismal dilatation of the right renal artery. (c) Super-selective renal arteriography discriminates between renal artery and aneurismal dilatation. (d) Renal venogram shows the direct communication between renal vein and anueurysmal dilatation. Therefore, aneurismal dilatation of the renal vein could be induced by arterialization of the renal vein due to arteriovenous fistula. (e), (f) After coil embolization of renal arteriovenous fistula with microcoils, the renal AVF disappeared.

http://dx.doi.org/10.5772/56730

3.8. Pelvic AVFs (Fig.9)

Pelvic AVF is rare. It is also difficult to manage or control it. Because it may have numerous and complex vessels, embolotherapy via the arterial side has a limitation to occlude the nidus. Do et al. [26] reported high complete regression rate (83.3%) by arterial ethanol embolotherapy combined with venous coil embolization. A case was reported whose pelvic AVF was successfully treated by venous embolization under balloon occlusion [27]. This technique is usually used for treatment of gastric varices and portal hypertension [28].

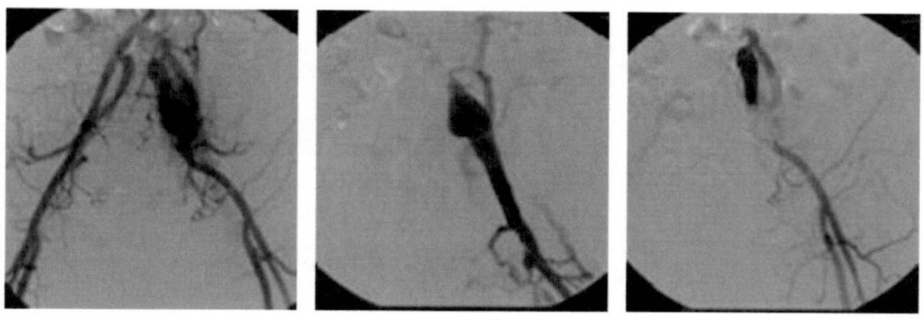

(a) (b) (c)

Figure 9. Pelvic AVMs. (a) Aortography shows fine vessels proliferation around the left iliac artery and subsequent early visualization of left iliac veins. (b)Venography shows occlusion of the left common iliac vein. (c)Fine vessels proliferation and early venous drainage are not observed by left common iliac arteriography.

3.9. Uterine AVMs (Fig.10)

The etiology of uterine AVFs covers a wide spectrum including iatrogenic and post dilate and curettage ones, vascular tumor, and trophoblastic disease [29]. Like other organ involved AVMs, controlling the blood flow of the nidus is difficult and surgical intervention (hysterectomy) is dangerous because intraoperative bleeding is tremendous [30]. Selective arterial embolotherapy is useful in some uterine AVMs cases, but we experienced an unsuccessful case of uterine AVMs that substituted for operative uterine artery clamping [31].

3.10. Upper and lower extremity AVMs

AVMs of the upper and lower extremities may manifest cosmetic distortion and painful tumor. Besides them, venous hypertension due to peripheral AVMs leads to bony osteolysis and distortion, sometimes results in pathological fracture. Do et al [32] have reported that patients with peripheral subcutaneous AVMs have the bone involvement in 59% of the patients. For the management of residual subcutaneous AVMs, the authors have recommended that patients wear compression stockings rather than undergo additional ethanol embolotherapy, which can result in skin necrosis [32]. In addition, as mentioned previously [16], ablation of the AVMs require stasis of absolute ethanol within not only the nidus but also angiopathic feeding or drainage vessels.

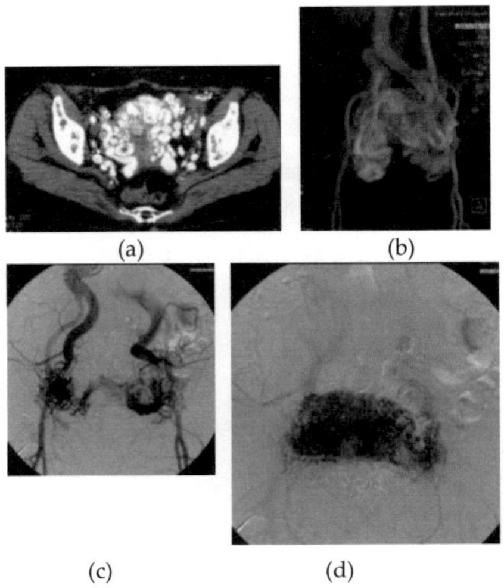

Figure 10. Uterine AVMs. Tortuous and dilated vessels are present in the entire uterus on contrast enhanced CT (a) and magnetic resonance arteriography (b). Pelvic arteriograms (c, d) show numerous and tortuous dilated vessels throughout the uterus ad early venous drainage. Reproduced from reference [31] with the permission of the publisher.

3.11. Lower extremity AVFs with DVT (Deep Vein Thrombosis) (Fig.11)

Venous obstruction mainly due to venous thrombosis is an underlying cause of phleboid disease [33-35]. However, reports of AVF in the leg are rare, and no guidelines have been developed for the treatment of AVFs in the leg [36,37]. Deep-vein thrombosis may be followed by Inflammation and neovascularity to form AVFs. First, low oxygenation due to thrombogenesis and various vascular growth factors increase the venous pressure. Chemical factors are then released by the vascular endothelium, vasa vasorum, and platelets to initiate the inflammatory process. Next, neovascularization induces thrombotic reconstitution and activates various inflammatory cells [37]. We therefore recommend restoring the venous occlusion before performing arterial embolization in patients with both AVF and venous occlusion.

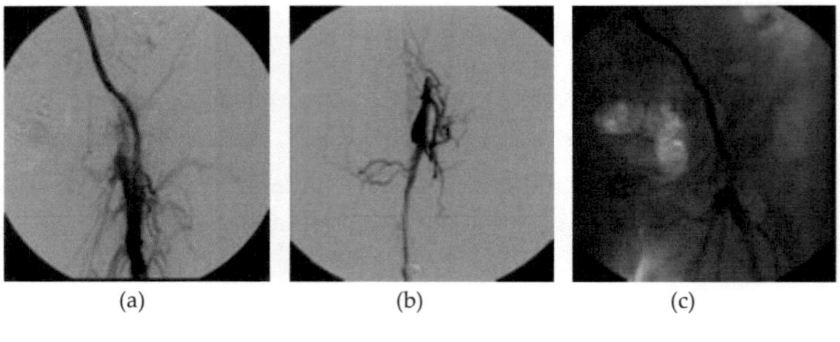

Figure 11. Leg AVFs with deep vein thrombosis. (a) Aortography shows fine vessels proliferation around the left internal iliac artery and early visualization of the left iliac vein. (b)Venography shows occlusion of the left common iliac vein. (c)After balloon PTA and stent deployment, venography shows recanalization of the left common iliac vein.

4. Conclusion

Endovascular therapy including embolotherapy, sclerotherapy or their combination could be an option for treating a patient with AVM (AVF), because complete resectability of AVMs is low. According to the location of AVMs, flow speed of the nidus and relation with other organs, appropriate embolic and sclerotic materials should be chosen to obtain good clinical outcome.

Author details

Yasutaka Baba*, Sadao Hayashi and Masayuki Nakajo

*Address all correspondence to: yasutaka@m3.kufm.kagoshima-u.ac.jp

Department of Radiology, Kagoshima University, Sakuragaoka, Kagoshima-shi, Kagoshima, Japan

References

[1] Odile Enjolras MWaRC. Introduction: ISSVA Classification. London: Cambridge University Press; 2007,pp 2-11.

[2] Lacout A, Marcy PY, Thariat J, El Hajjam M, Lacombe P. VEGF target in HHT lung patients: the role of bevacizumab as a possible alternative to embolization. Med Hypotheses. 2012; May;78(5) 689-90.

[3] Giordano P, Lenato GM, Pierucci P, Suppressa P, Altomare M, Del Vecchio G, et al. Effects of VEGF on phenotypic severity in children with hereditary hemorrhagic telangiectasia. J Pediatr Hematol Oncol. 2009; Aug;31(8) 577-582.

[4] Sabba C, Pasculli G, Lenato GM, Suppressa P, Lastella P, Memeo M, et al. Hereditary hemorrhagic telangiectasia: clinical features in ENG and ALK1 mutation carriers. J Thromb Haemost. 2007; Jun;5(6) 1149-1157.

[5] McDonald J, Pyeritz RE. Hereditary Hemorrhagic Telangiectasia. In: Pagon RA, Bird TD, Dolan CR, Stephens K, Adam MP. (ed.) Gene Reviews ™ [Internet]. Seattle (WA): University of Washington, Seattle; 1993-.2000 Jun 26 [updated 2012 Jan 05] http://www.ncbi.nlm.nih.gov/books/NBK1351/

[6] Dupuis-Girod S, Ginon I, Saurin JC, Marion D, Guillot E, Decullier E, et al. Bevacizumab in patients with hereditary hemorrhagic telangiectasia and severe hepatic vascular malformations and high cardiac output. JAMA. 2012; Mar 7;307(9) 948-955.

[7] Remy-Jardin M, Dumont P, Brillet PY, Dupuis P, Duhamel A, Remy J. Pulmonary arteriovenous malformations treated with embolotherapy: helical CT evaluation of

long-term effectiveness after 2-21-year follow-up. Radiology. 2006; May;239(2) 576-585.

[8] Pollak JS, Saluja S, Thabet A, Henderson KJ, Denbow N, White RI, Jr. Clinical and anatomic outcomes after embolotherapy of pulmonary arteriovenous malformations. J Vasc Interv Radiol. 2006; Jan;17(1) 35-44.

[9] White RI, Jr., Lynch-Nyhan A, Terry P, Buescher PC, Farmlett EJ, Charnas L, et al. Pulmonary arteriovenous malformations: techniques and long-term outcome of embolotherapy. Radiology. 1988; Dec;169(3) 663-669.

[10] Mathis S, Dupuis-Girod S, Plauchu H, Giroud M, Barroso B, Ly KH, et al. Cerebral abscesses in hereditary haemorrhagic telangiectasia: a clinical and microbiological evaluation. Clin Neurol Neurosurg. 2011; Apr;114(3) 235-240.

[11] Lee DW, White RI, Jr., Egglin TK, Pollak JS, Fayad PB, Wirth JA, et al. Embolotherapy of large pulmonary arteriovenous malformations: long-term results. Ann Thorac Surg. 1997; Oct;64(4) 930-939; discussion 9-40.

[12] Cil B, Canyigit M, Ozkan OS, Pamuk GA, Dogan R. Bilateral multiple pulmonary arteriovenous malformations: endovascular treatment with the Amplatzer Vascular Plug. J Vasc Interv Radiol. 2006; Jan;17(1) 141-145.

[13] Sagara K, Miyazono N, Inoue H, Ueno K, Nishida H, Nakajo M. Recanalization after coil embolotherapy of pulmonary arteriovenous malformations: study of long-term outcome and mechanism for recanalization. AJR Am J Roentgenol. 1998; Mar;170(3) 727-730.

[14] Grillo HC, Athanasoulis CA. Tracheal obstruction from mediastinal arteriovenous malformation. J Thorac Cardiovasc Surg. 2004; Nov;128(5) 780-782.

[15] Pekkola J, Lappalainen K, Vuola P, Klockars T, Salminen P, Pitkaranta A. Head and Neck Arteriovenous Malformations: Results of Ethanol Sclerotherapy. AJNR Am J Neuroradiol. 2012; Jul 5. [Epub ahead of print]

[16] Baba Y, Miyazono N, Kanetsuki I, Nishi H, Hamada H, Nakajo M. Re: Combined arteriovenous malformation and aneurysm of the ulnar artery: successful arterial embolization by using absolute ethanol. Cardiovasc Intervent Radiol. 1999; May-Jun; 22(3) 266-267.

[17] Baba Y, Ohkubo K, Hamada K, Hokotate H, Nakajo M. Hyperintense basal ganglia lesions on T1-weighted images in hereditary hemorrhagic telangiectasia with hepatic involvement. J Comput Assist Tomogr. 1998; Nov-Dec;22(6) 976-979.

[18] Senokuchi T, Baba Y, Hayashi S, Nakajo M. Embolization of hepatic arteriovenous shunt with absolute ethanol in a patient with hepatocellular carcinoma. Cardiovasc Intervent Radiol.2010; Feb;34 Suppl 2 S154-156.

[19] Hayashi S, Baba Y, Ueno K, Nakajo M. Small arteriovenous malformation of the common bile duct causing hemobilia in a patient with hereditary hemorrhagic telangiectasia. Cardiovasc Intervent Radiol. 2008; Jul 31 Suppl 2 S131-134.

[20] Barth MM, Khwaja K, Faintuch S, Rabkin D. Transarterial and transvenous embolotherapy of arteriovenous fistulas in the transplanted pancreas. J Vasc Interv Radiol. 2008; Aug;19(8) 1231-1235.

[21] Defreyne L, Verstraeten V, De Potter C, Pattyn P, De Vos M, Kunnen M. Jejunal arteriovenous malformation, diagnosed by angiography and treated by embolization and catheter-guided surgery: case report and review of literature. Abdom Imaging. 1998; Mar-Apr;23(2) 127-131.

[22] Gordhan AD, Newey CR, Wong G, Wieland J. N-butyl cyanoacrylate embolization of small bowel arteriovenous malformation presenting with acute massive lower gastrointestinal hemorrhage. J Vasc Interv Radiol. 2008; Nov;19(11) 1669-1670.

[23] Liao Z, Gao R, Li ZS. Vascular malformation of the small intestine. Endoscopy. 2007; Feb;39 Suppl 1:E319.

[24] Uthoff H, Pena C, Contreras F, Katzen BT. Symptomatic ascites caused by a longstanding posttraumatic mesenteric arteriovenous fistula. J Vasc Interv Radiol.2012; May; 23(5) 722-724.

[25] Cura M, Elmerhi F, Suri R, Bugnone A, Dalsaso T. Vascular malformations and arteriovenous fistulas of the kidney. Acta Radiol. 2010; Mar;51(2) 144-149.

[26] Do YS, Kim YW, Park KB, Kim DI, Park HS, Cho SK, et al. Endovascular treatment combined with emboloscleorotherapy for pelvic arteriovenous malformations. J Vasc Surg. 2011; Feb;55(2) 465-471.

[27] Mitsuzaki K, Yamashita Y, Utsunomiya D, Sumi S, Ogata I, Takahashi M, et al. Balloon-occluded retrograde transvenous embolization of a pelvic arteriovenous malformation. Cardiovasc Intervent Radiol. 1999; Nov-Dec;22(6) 518-520.

[28] Kanekawa H, Kayama A, Goto K, Kawanishi T, Yamazaki T, Mima S. [Balloon-occluded retrograde transvenous obliteration for treatment of gastroesophageal varices]. Nihon Geka Gakkai Zasshi. 1996; Jan;97(1) 78-82.

[29] Kwon JH, Kim GS. Obstetric iatrogenic arterial injuries of the uterus: diagnosis with US and treatment with transcatheter arterial embolization. Radiographics. 2002; Jan-Feb;22(1) 35-46.

[30] Cura M, Martinez N, Cura A, Dalsaso TJ, Elmerhi F. Arteriovenous malformations of the uterus. Acta Radiol. 2009; Sep;50(7) 823-829.

[31] Yokomine D, Yoshinaga M, Baba Y, Matsuo T, Iguro Y, Nakajo M, et al. Successful management of uterine arteriovenous malformation by ligation of feeding artery af-

ter unsuccessful uterine artery embolization. J Obstet Gynaecol Res. 2009; Feb;35(1) 183-188.

[32] Do YS, Park KB, Park HS, Cho SK, Shin SW, Moon JW, et al. Extremity arteriovenous malformations involving the bone: therapeutic outcomes of ethanol embolotherapy. J Vasc Interv Radiol. 2010; Jun;21(6) 807-816.

[33] Fournier D, Rodesch G, Terbrugge K, Flodmark O, Lasjaunias P. Acquired mural (dural) arteriovenous shunts of the vein of Galen. Report of 4 cases. Neuroradiology. 1991; 33(1) 52-55.

[34] Ozawa T, Miyasaka Y, Tanaka R, Kurata A, Fujii K. Dural-pial arteriovenous malformation after sinus thrombosis. Stroke. 1998; Aug;29(8) 1721-1724.

[35] Phatouros CC, Halbach VV, Dowd CF, Lempert TE, Malek AM, Meyers PM, et al. Acquired pial arteriovenous fistula following cerebral vein thrombosis. Stroke. 1999; Nov;30(11) 2487-2490.

[36] Link DP, Garza AS, Monsky W. Acquired peripheral arteriovenous malformations in patients with venous thrombosis: report of two cases. J Vasc Interv Radiol. 2010; Mar; 21(3) 387-391.

[37] Labropoulos N, Bhatti AF, Amaral S, Leon L, Borge M, Rodriguez H, et al. Neovascularization in acute venous thrombosis. J Vasc Surg. 2005; Sep;42(3) 515-518.

Chapter 8

Ultrasound Guided Non Surgical Closure of Post Angiographic Femoral Arteriovenous Fistula (AVF) and Pseudoaneurysm (PSA)

Akram M. Asbeutah, Pushpinder S. Khera and Abdullah Ramadan

Additional information is available at the end of the chapter

http://dx.doi.org/10.5772/55835

1. Introduction

1.1. Indications for AVF treatment

Local complications of femoral arterial catheterization like hematomas, pseudoaneurysm (PSA) and arteriovenous fistula (AVF) are increasing in incidence due to the large number of patients undergoing diagnostic and therapeutic angiographic procedures through this route [1 - 3] (see figure 1). A PSA refers to a confined collection of thrombus and blood associated with tear of one or more layers of an arterial wall [4]. An iatrogenic AVF occurs when an arterial puncture inadvertently extends to involve an adjacent vein leading to a communication between the two. Color flow Doppler ultrasound is the imaging modality of choice for the diagnosis and assessment of a PSA, with a high sensitivity and specificity [5].

Incidence of post-angiographic femoral PSA and AVF varies between 0.07-9% [1], [6]. The risk factors include age more than 65 years, low or high femoral arterial puncture, anticoagulation and use of a large arterial sheath size [7].

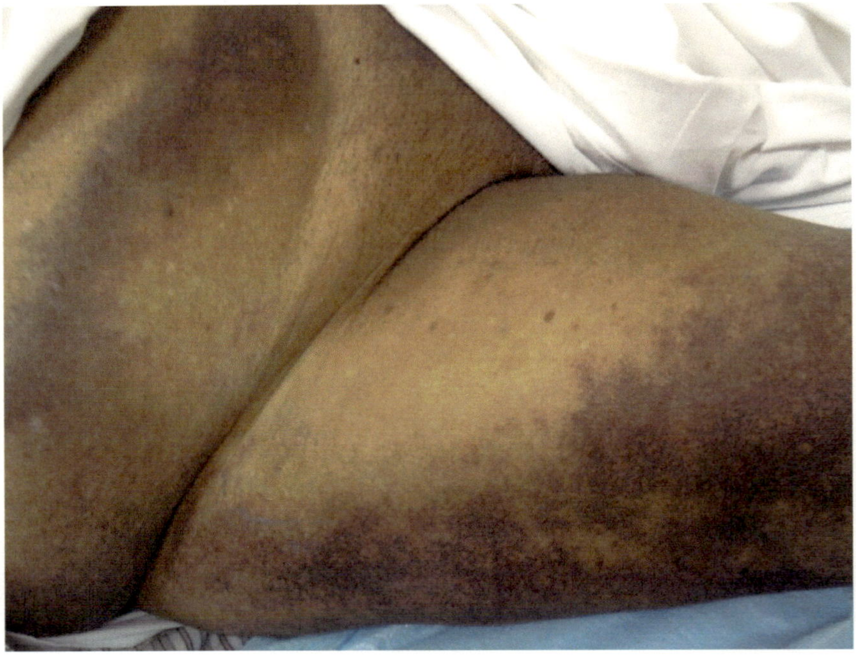

Figure 1. Ecchymosis of the right thigh and lower abdominal wall.

2. AFV diagnosis using imaging modalities

In the femoral region, turbulence is seen within either the common femoral or profunda femoral vein with arterialized signals shown on the Doppler spectrum (see Figure 2A). The fistulous communication can be seen on color flow Doppler, although it may be difficult to localize with duplex ultrasound alone (see Figure 2B). The turbulence associated with the fistula can be confused with turbulent signals due to extrinsic compression of the vein by hematoma or PSA, which is also a common complication following catheterization. The characteristic findings of a PSA include a slow swirling flow [Yin -Yang sign] within a hypoechoic lesion which is connected to the parent artery via a neck (see Figure 3 A-D). The latter displays a characteristic "to-and-fro" high velocity flow [4]. Doppler features of an AVF include a region of aliasing interposed between an artery and vein with increased diastolic flow in the artery and turbulent flow within the vein [8].

Visualization of the communicating channel allows a confident diagnosis of AVF rather than extrinsic venous compression by the surrounding hematoma or PSA. The use of computerized axial tomography (CTA) can resolve the problem (see Figure 4 A-B).

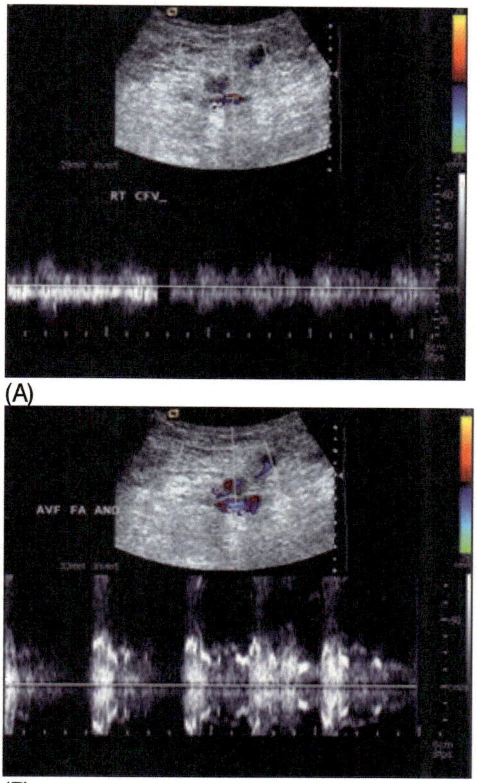

(A)

(B)

Figure 2. (A) Color Doppler image depicts arterial signals within the FV waveform indicating an arterio-venous communication; (B) Color Doppler image showing turbulent waveform within the AV fistula.

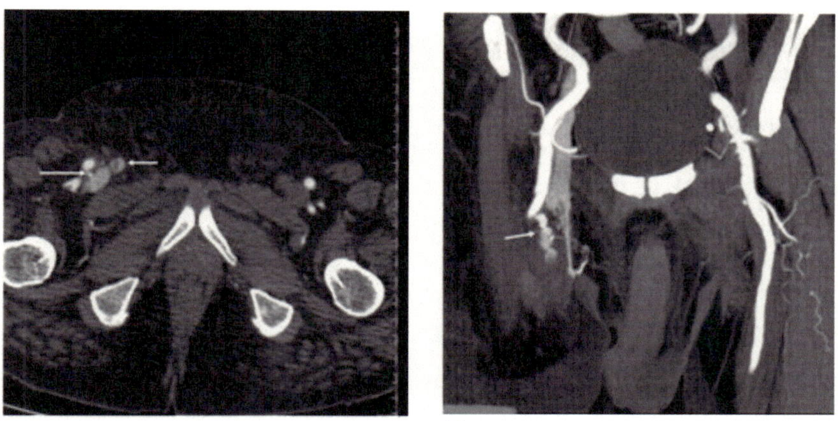

(A) (B)

Figure 4. (A) CT angiography axial image depicts a thin linear communication (long arrow) between the posterior wall of FA and FV with opacification of the latter and the proximal great saphenous vein (short arrow); and (B) Coronal

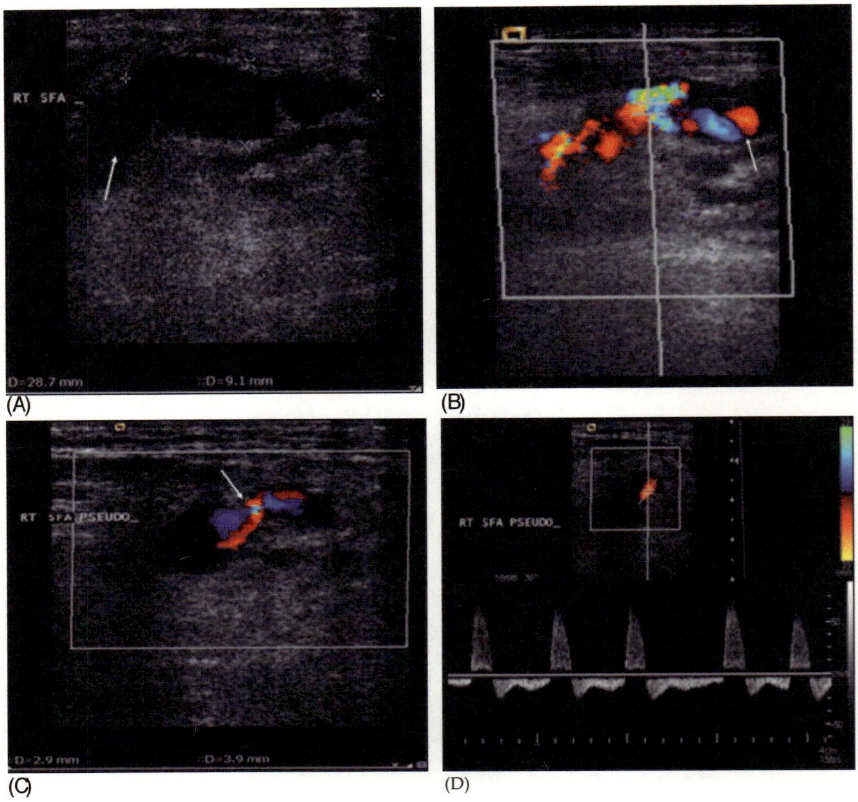

Figure 3. (A) Grey scale image showing the pseudoaneurysm as an oblong sonolucent structure anterior to the right FA (arrow); (B) Color Doppler image shows swirling flow within it the" Yin -Yang sign" (arrow); C) The connection (neck) between the FA and PSA (arrow); and (D) Pulsed wave Doppler image of the PSA neck depicts to-and-fro flow within it.

reformatted image showing the PSA (arrow) arising from the FA. The CFV and the external iliac veins are opacified due to presence of the AV fistula.

3. Methods of treatment for AVF

Transcutaneous therapy aimed at achieving closure of the fistula has been described using ultrasound monitoring and by applying pressure over the fistula for periods of 20 to 60 minutes success rates are 30% or lower [12].

Despite ultrasound guided thrombin injection [UGTI] is an off label use of topical thrombin which is not FDA approved for injection, but it is only the treatment of choice when favorable anatomy is present such as a well defined narrow neck for post catheterization PSA [5 - 7]. Ultrasound guided compression [USGC] without thrombin injection retains a high success rate [6, 7] and it is a useful substitute for inducing thrombosis in the PSA and closure of AVF tract, with good results [10-17]

4. Treatment algorithm for AVF

Any patient who experiences local site pain disproportionate to that expected after an angiographic procedure should be evaluated with duplex ultrasound to rule out the presence of a PSA and/or AVF. Color Doppler ultrasound and spectral analysis has a high sensitivity [94%] and specificity [97%] for detection of a PSA [4].

Untreated PSA can lead to progressive lesion enlargement, infection, compression neuropathy and rupture [12]. Until the early nineties, surgery was the only treatment available for PSA and AVF closure. Presently it is only rarely employed to treat the post catheterisation PSA, when other treatment options fail or if a complication develops [13].

In 1991 Fellmeth et al. described a method of ultrasound guided compression (USGC) for closing post catheterization femoral PSA and AVF [12]. Subsequent studies confirmed a high rate of success [varying from 75% to >90%] for closure of PSA by this method [14 - 15]. In patients on anticoagulants, the success rate is reported to be between 30%-73 % [14 - 17]. Success rate for AVF closure is described between 33%-50% [12 - 16].

The mechanical compression is exerted using the ultrasound probe and is positioned directly over the neck of the PSA or the tract in case of the AVF [12]. It is titrated so as to obliterate blood flow within them. At all times an adequate flow is maintained in the concerned artery. The compression is usually continued for cycles of 10 minutes each with intermittent release to assess for closure of the neck. This can be repeated till the neck is closed or else discontinued if the physician/patient develops fatigue [13].

The only limiting factor in USGC method is the time it takes to induce thrombosis to close the PSA or AVF tract [13]. Patient may experience intra-procedural pain which responds to intravenous analgesia [12]. Complications are rare and include vasovagal reactions, PSA rupture, skin necrosis and DVT [13].

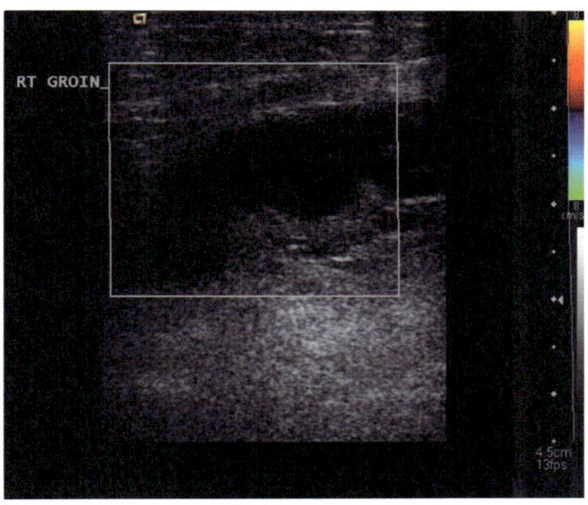

Figure 5. Successful post compression thrombosis of the PSA &AVF.

Successful obliteration o the PSA and the AVF is the main goal of the whole procedure (see Figure 5). This is the major goal every treating physician should achieve for better patient management and treatment.

Ultrasound guided compression of the post-angiographic femoral arterial injuries is a technically simple and relatively safe method.

Author details

Akram M. Asbeutah[1*], Pushpinder S. Khera[2] and Abdullah Ramadan[2]

*Address all correspondence to: asbeutah_akram@hotmail.com or akram.asbeutah@hsc.edu.kw

1 Department of Radiologic Sciences, Faculty of Allied Health Sciences, Kuwait University, Sulaibekhat, Kuwait

2 Department of Radiology, Al-Sabah Hospital, Ministry of Health, Kuwait

References

[1] Babu, S. C, Piccorelli, G. O, Shah, P. M, Stein, J. H, & Clauss, R. H. Incidence and results of arterial complications among 16,350 patients undergoing cardiac catheterization. J Vasc Surg (1989). , 10, 113-16.

[2] Glaser, R. L, Mckellar, D, & Scher, K. S. Arterio-venous fistulas after cardiac catheterization. Arch Surg (1989). , 124, 1313-15.

[3] Bourassa, M. G, & Noble, J. Complication rate of coronary arteriography: a review of 5250 cases by percutaneous femoral technique. Circulation (1976). , 53, 106-14.

[4] Burke, B. J, & Friedman, S. G. Ultrasound in the diagnosis and management of arterial emergencies. In, Zwiebel WJ(ed). Introduction to vascular ultrasonography, 5th edition. Philadelphia, Elsevier Saunders,(2005). , 381-99.

[5] Coughlin, B. F, & Paushter, D. M. Peripheral pseudoaneurysms: evaluation with duplex US. Radiology (1988). , 168, 339-42.

[6] Kresowik, T. F, Khoury, M. D, Miller, B. V, Winniford, M. D, Shamma, A. R, Sharp, W. J, et al. A prospective study of the incidence and natural history of femoral vascular complications after percutaneous transluminal coronary angioplasty. J Vasc Surg (1991). , 13, 328-336.

[7] Morgan, R, & Belli, A. M. Current treatment methods for postcatheterization pseudoaneurysms. J Vasc Interv Radiol (2003). , 14, 697-710.

[8] La Perna LOlin JW, Goines D, Childs MB, Ouriel K. Ultrasound-guided thrombin injection for the treatment of postcatheterization pseudoaneurysms. Circulation (2000). , 102, 2391-95.

[9] Taylor, B. S, Rhee, R. Y, Muluk, S, Trachtenberg, J, Walters, D, Steed, D. L, et al. Thrombin injection versus compression of femoral artery pseudoaneurysms. J Vacs Surg (1999). , 30, 1052-59.

[10] Weinmann, E. E, Chayen, D, Kobzantev, Z. V, Zaretsky, M, & Bass, A. Treatment of postcatheterisation false aneurysms: ultrasound-guided compression vs ultrasound-guided thrombin injection. Eur J Vasc Endovasc Surg (2002). , 23, 68-72.

[11] Altstidi, R, Lehmkuhl, H. B, Voss, E, Herold, C, Becker, D, Giinter, E, et al. Ultrasound-guided nonsurgical closure of postangiographic femoral artery injuries. Vasc Endovascular Surg (1997). , 31, 781-90.

[12] Fellmeth, B. D, Roberts, A. C, Bookstein, J. J, Freischlag, J. A, Forsythe, J. R, Buckner, N. K, et al. Postangiographic femoral artery injuries: nonsurgical repair with US-guided compression. Radiology (1991). , 178, 671-675.

[13] Webber, G. W, Jang, J, Gustavson, S, & Olin, J. W. Contemporary management of postcatheterization pseudoaneurysms. Circulation (2007). , 115, 2666-74.

[14] Eisenberg, L, Paulson, E. K, Kliewer, M. A, Hudson, M. P, Delong, D. M, & Carroll, B. A. Sonographically guided compression repair of pseudoaneurysms: further experience from a single institution. Am J Roentgenol (1999). , 173, 1567-73.

[15] Steinkamp, H. J, Werk, M, & Felix, R. Treatment of postinterventional pseudoaneurysms by ultrasound-guided compression. Invest Radiol (2000). , 35, 186-92.

[16] Schaub, F, Theiss, W, Heinz, M, Zagel, M, & Schomig, A. New aspects in ultrasound-guided compression repair of post-catheterization femoral artery injuries. Circulation (1994). , 90, 1861-65.

[17] Dean, S. M, Olin, J. W, Piedmonte, M, Grubb, M, & Young, J. R. Ultrasound guided compression closure of postcatheterization pseudoaneurysms during concurrent anticoagulation: a review of seventy-seven patients. J Vasc surg (1996). , 23, 28-34.

Chapter 9

Role of Collateral Vein Occlusion in Autologous Dysfunctional Hemodialysis Fistulas

Iftikhar Ahmad

Additional information is available at the end of the chapter

http://dx.doi.org/10.5772/56462

1. Introduction

An autologous arterial-venous fistula is the most desirable vascular access for end-stage renal disease (ESRD) patients who are dependent on hemodialysis. [1] Autologous arterial-venous fistulas have a lower risk of thrombosis and infection, and have shown to have a longer patency as well. [1] Kidney Dialysis Outline and Quality Initiative (KDOQI) guidelines mandate that 50% of all new hemodialysis accesses and 40% of all hemodialysis accesses be autologous arterial-venous fistulas.

Unfortunately, not all fistulas mature enough to be used for hemodialysis. The failure rate of a fistula to mature in the earlier studies ranged from 10%-55%. [2,3] As the mean survival age of hemodialysis patients has increased, surgeons are creating fistulas in elderly patients with less than ideal vessels, thereby increasing the rate of non-maturing fistulas and reducing their long-term patency. The later studies have shown a significant increase in the number of native fistulas failing to reach maturity without intervention. [4-9]

The Fistula First initiative has made a concerted effort to increase the number of patients on hemodialysis to have autologous fistulas rather than synthetic grafts or tunneled hemodialysis catheters. An increase in the number of native fistulas has also created an unintended consequence of a higher number of these fistulas not reaching maturation. [10] Aggressive early intervention in a non-maturing autologous arterial-venous fistula results in a high percentage of these fistulas reaching maturation. [9]

The two most common causes of non-maturing and mal-functioning autologous fistulas are anastomotic and juxta-anastomotic stenoses reducing the blood flow through the outflow vein and collateral veins which drain part of the blood away from the main outflow vein, thereby making the volume of blood flow in the main outflow vein suboptimal for hemodialysis. [11]

Anastomotic or juxta-anastomotic stenosis is the most common cause of a fistula failing to mature. The stenosis most likely occurs because of operative trauma. In case of transposed vein fistulas, the loss of vasa vasorum in the mobilized portion of the vein may also contribute to causation of stenosis. Secondly, there is element of neo-intimal hyperplasia. Because of the large pressure gradient between arterial and venous circulation, the blood accelerates while passing from the artery to the vein causing turbulent flow that is considered responsible for endothelial damage as a result of micro trauma.

The role of preventing blood flow through the competing accessory or collateral veins by embolization or ligation is questionable. [1] There are no prospective studies which evaluate the effect of embolization or ligation of the collaterals on fistula maturation or patency.

In this chapter, the approach to treating non-maturing fistulas will be discussed as it applies to the embolization of competing collaterals.

2. Rationale

Traditional surgical practice has been to abandon autologous arteriovenous fistulas that fail to mature in three to four months in favor of a new fistula, or a graft. Recently however, there has been a drive to intervene aggressively on the non-maturing fistulas to assist them to mature.

With advances in medicine and better healthcare delivery, life spans of patients on hemodialysis are increasing and these patients are outliving their hemodialysis access sites. There are only a finite number of sites in a patient suitable for access creation. As these fistulas fail and are abandoned in favor of new ones, the patients eventually run out of options for access sites. It is therefore imperative for physicians responsible for maintaining these accesses to treat these fistulas aggressively to maintain their patency for as long as possible in order to maximize the patients' life expectancy.

The role of angioplasty of anastomotic or juxta-anastomotic stenosis in assisting non-maturing fistulas to reach maturity is well documented. [1,2] Tessitore et al. demonstrated in their landmark prospective study that even in the absence of hemodynamic blood flow abnormality, preemptive angioplasty of the anastomotic and juxta-anastomotic stenosis leads to a four-fold increase in the median survival of the fistula and almost a three-fold decrease in the risk of their failure.

The role of collateral vein embolization, however, is less well established. Intuitively, and hemodynamically, it makes sense to maximize blood flow through a single outflow vein, thereby providing adequate flow for hemodialysis. If there are competing parallel outflow veins for which there is a single inflow artery of a finite size, the flow through individual venous channel will decrease despite the overall decrease in the resistance offered by multiple parallel channels. The parallel outflow veins, which have different calibers, lengths, tortuosity, and flow patterns, further complicate the flow dynamics (Figure 1).

(a)

(b)

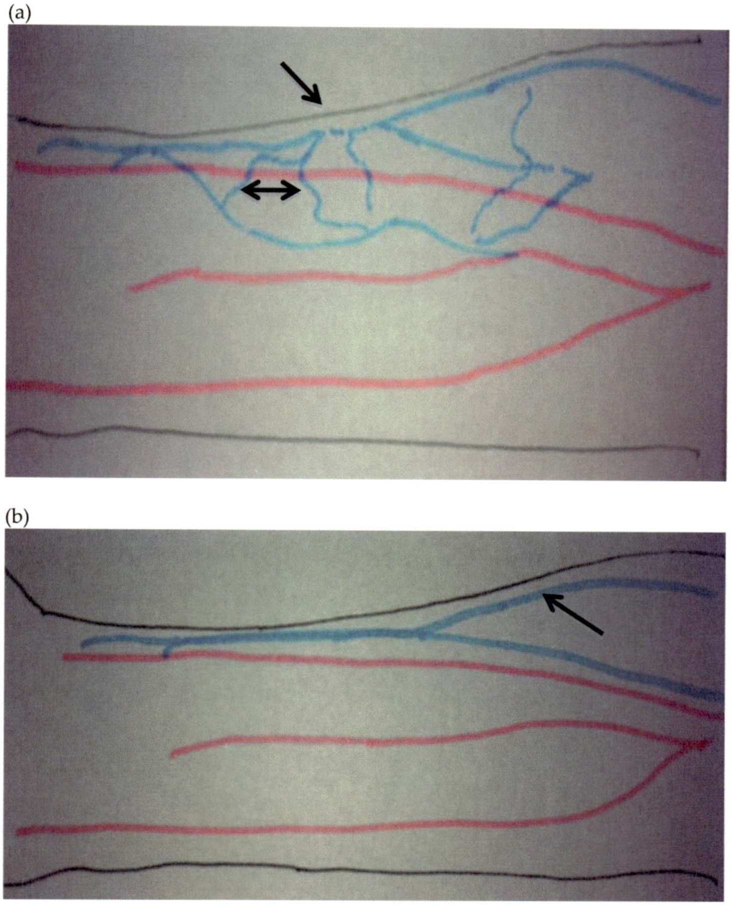

Figure 1. Demonstrates schematic diagram of a radial artery to cephalic venous fistula demonstrating multiple collaterals (double headed arrow in figure 1 a) due to a tight stenosis in the cephalic outflow vein (single headed arrow in figure 1 a). After treatment of the culprit stenosis, there is single inline flow in the main cephalic vein (single headed arrow in figure 1 b) and no further filling of the collaterals.

Arterial inflow increases in response to decreased resistance in the venous outflow. In most cases, arterial inflow is insufficient to sustain adequate outflow through each collateral channel to for adequate hemodialysis.

3. Technique

It is best to approach a non-maturing autologous arterial-venous fistula, by obtaining a detailed history of hemodialysis access, in particular, as it pertains to the access in question. This should be followed by a thorough physical examination of the fistula. The physical exam can reveal much of what one might expect on fistulogram. Robbin et al. have shown that experienced operators on physical examination alone can predict with 80% accuracy if the fistula will mature. [12]

Physical examination can reveal the cause of the underlying anatomical abnormality quite accurately. [13] In a normally developed fistula, there is a continuous thrill from the anastomosis all the way centrally along the outflow vein. The thrill gradually decreases in intensity from the anastomosis centrally. When patients have a critical stenosis in the outflow vein, the physical examination often reveals a strong pulse peripheral to the stenosis and a weak thrill centrally in the outflow vein. The pulse often has a water hammer character. [14] In the absence of a stenosis, the pulse is soft and easily compressible. The presence of collaterals can also be determined by physical examination. Compression of the outflow vein abolishes the thrill at the anastomotic site and converts it into a strong pulse. But if competing collaterals are present, the thrill persists even after compression of the main outflow vein, as blood continues to flow through the collateral. In addition, the character of the thrill changes central to the point of takeoff of the collateral veins. The thrill becomes significantly weaker and difficult to palpate.

The next step in approaching the non-maturing autologous hemodialysis fistula is to perform an ultrasound. This helps to confirm the findings of the physical examination. It also provides an idea as to the best site to puncture the fistula for intervention. Not infrequently, the arteriovenous anastomosis is difficult to identify because of severe anastomotic stenosis or because of a number of collateral venous channels close to the anastomosis stealing the blood from the main outflow. In these cases a reflux fistulogram is non-diagnostic as all the collateral veins fill up without correctly identifying the arteriovenous anastomosis. In these cases, it becomes imperative to puncture the brachial artery in the mid upper arm and perform an angiogram to identify the arterial-venous anastomosis. (Figure 2) The author restricts brachial artery access to a 3F inner dilator of the micro-puncture set. The arteriogram only serves the purpose of identifying the arteriovenous anastomosis. A retrograde puncture of the outflow vein is also needed in these cases, as all interventions are performed from the retrograde venous access in order to avoid a large caliber hole in the brachial artery.

The author initially identifies all the areas of stenosis and competing collateral veins by initial fistulogram. The stenosis responsible for non-maturation of the fistula is then treated with an appropriate size balloon angioplasty. Once the anastomosis is treated, the a fistulogram is performed with the catheter placed in the inflow artery to identify the result of angioplasty and whether the collaterals still fill. It is imperative that the fistulogram both before and after angioplasty of the stenotic lesion be performed with the catheter tip in the inflow artery, and not by means of a reflux fistulogram by occluding the outflow vein. If the fistulogram is performed using the reflux technique, the collaterals are likely to appear more prominent than they actually are.

The fistulogram is then reviewed in conjunction with the clinical exam. If the post angioplasty fistulogram and the clinical exam indicate that there has been no significant decrease in the filling of the collaterals, occlusion of the blood flow through the collaterals is indicated. (Figure 3) The occlusion of the blood flow in the collaterals is performed either by embolization or surgical ligation of the vein.

http://dx.doi.org/10.5772/56462

a

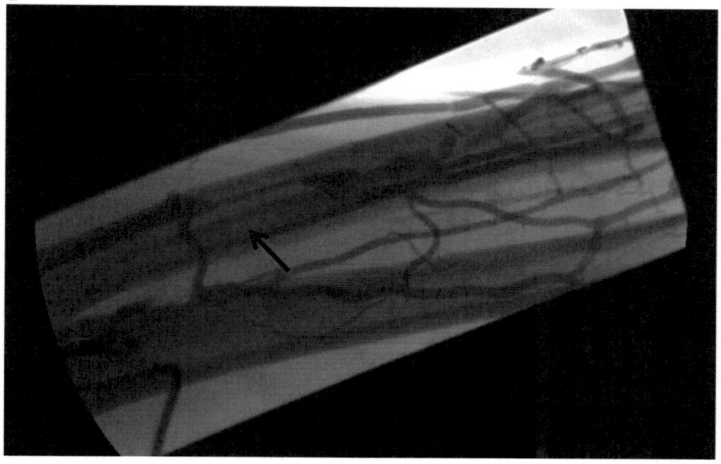

b

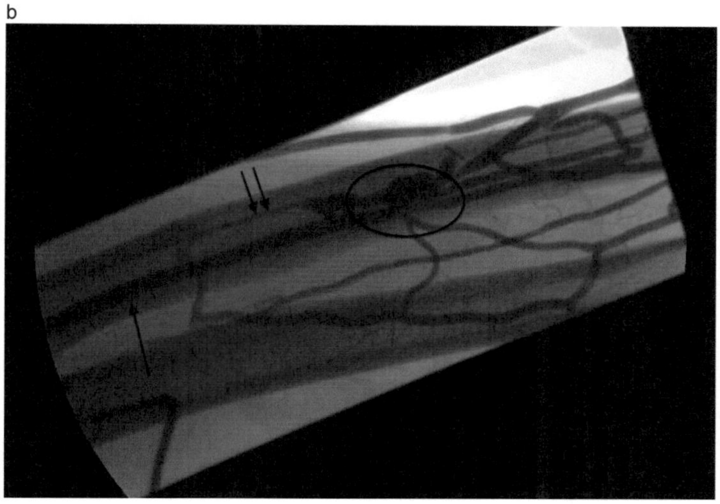

Figure 2. Demonstrates reflux injection of contrast through the cephalic outflow vein in the forearm (single arrow in figure 2 a), which fails to demonstrate the arteriovenous anastomosis. The injection however, fills multiple collaterals. The reason for this occurrence is that reflux injection of contrast encounters un-opacified blood flowing in through the artery and because of the stenosis; the injection pressure is generally unable to get reflux into the artery. There is greater opacification of collaterals for same reason. Figure 2 b shows injection through the brachial artery (single long arrow in figure 2 b), which clearly demonstrates the arteriovenous anastomosis (oval in figure 2 b) with retrograde filling of multiple collaterals due to long segment stenosis of the cephalic outflow vein (double arrow in figure 2 b)

For the collateral veins that are visible on the skin surface, ligation is possible either using a percutaneous or cut down technique. The author performs a percutaneous ligation of the vein using ultrasound guidance. A curved needle is passed deep to the vein under ultrasound guidance while the vein is being visualized in cross-section. A return pass is made superficial to the vein but deep to the skin exiting the needle close to the initial entry site thus placing a purse-string suture around the vein.

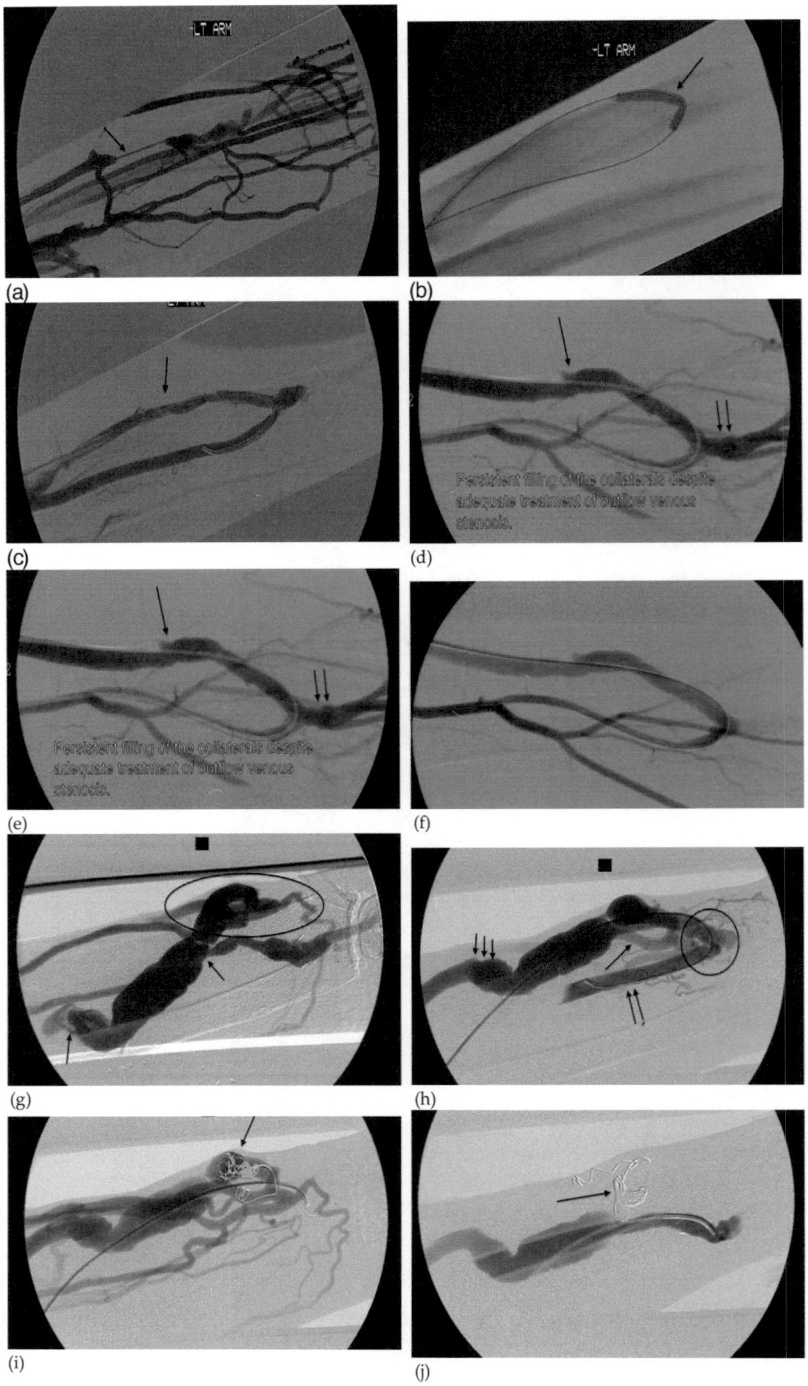

Figure 3. Reflux fistulogram on the same patient as in figure 2 demonstrates filling of multiple collaterals due to a long segment juxta-anastomotic stenosis (single arrow in figure 3 a). This lesion was successfully treated with angio-

plasty (single arrow in figure 3 b). Post angioplasty fistulogram showed no further filling of collaterals with inline flow through a single outflow vein, (single arrow in figure 3 c) which is significantly larger in caliber. In this case, the collateral veins were not embolized, as they did not fill in post angioplasty fistulogram. The second case demonstrated in figure 3 shows persistent filling of the competing veins in a patient who has a side-to-side radial artery to cephalic vein anastomosis. There is simultaneous filling of cephalic vein central and peripheral to the anastomosis (single arrow and double arrow respectively as seen in figure 3 d). In this case, the cephalic vein peripheral to the anastomosis was clearly visible on the skin, therefore, was ligated percutaneously using ultrasound guidance technique as described in the text. Follow-up fistulogram showed no further flow in the cephalic outflow vein peripheral to the anastomosis, and all the blood flowing centrally in the cephalic vein (figure 3 e) Third case shown in figure 3 demonstrates filling of multiple collaterals (oval in figure 3 f) due to two culprit stenoses (two separate single arrows in figure 3 f). Following successful treatment of these lesions with angioplasty, (triple arrows in figure 3 g) there was persistent filling of the collaterals (single arrow in figure 3 f). Since the collaterals were not clearly visible on the skin, they were treated with embolization using the technique described in the text (single arrow in figure 3 h). Post embolization completion fistulogram demonstrated inline flow in the main cephalic outflow vein without filling of the collaterals. Coils are seen occupying non-filling collaterals (figure 3 j)

If the competing collateral vein is not visible on the skin, it is embolized using regular 0.35 inch platform coils. The coils are oversized by about 20%-30%. The author's coil of preference is Tornado coil (large end first), which unfortunately is a special order item from Cook, Inc. (Cook Bloomington IN). Nester coil (Cook Bloomington IN) is also good; however, the Nester coil may prove more challenging to deploy for inexperienced operators. When fully deployed in the vessel, the Nester coil occupy a longer segment of the vein compared to a Tornado coil of the same size vein and coil combination. The collateral veins often have a short stump off the main outflow vein. In these cases precise coil deployment is important. Nester coils, on occasion, can be pushed too far into the collaterals, thereby blocking the blood flow in otherwise unintended veins. Additionally, because Nester coils occupy a longer segment of the vein, they tend to push the catheter tip back, if there is not enough purchase of the catheter tip within the collateral, which results in part of the coil protruding into the main outflow vein. In such a case, the coil will have to be retrieved by snare. The advantage of "large-end-first" Tornado coils over the "short-end-first" coils is that their deployment is more precise. The large end of the Tornado coil encounters the vessel wall immediately after coming out of the catheter tip, anchoring the coil to the vein wall. On the other hand, the short end of the "short-end-first" Tornado coils tends to float away from the catheter tip before the large end engages with the vessel wall to fixate the coil in the vessel.

4. Discussion

A significant number of native arteriovenous fistulas fail to mature [3-10]. Traditionally, the surgeons abandoned these fistulas in favor of new fistulas or synthetic grafts.

There are only a finite number of sites in the human body to create hemodialysis fistulas. All hemodialysis accesses fail at some point; as such, it is imperative for the interventionalist involved in maintaining the fistula to do everything possible within reason to keep each hemodialysis access patent for as long as possible. Keeping this in mind, interventionalists are now addressing non-maturing arteriovenous fistulas much more aggressively. [5-10]

Treatment of a native arteriovenous fistula entails angioplasty of arteriovenous anastomosis or juxta-anastomotic stenoses. [1,5-12] Although the role of angioplasty of swing point and juxtaanastomotic stenosis is quite clear, the role of collateral vein embolization or ligation remains controversial.

Maturation of the fistula involves adaptation of the vein walls to allow repeated punctures and increase in the blood pressure and flow. When the arteriovenous fistula is created, the high-pressure arterial blood is shunted into low-pressure veins. The thicker walls of the arteries can sustain the high arterial pressure, but the thin wall veins require some time to adapt to this high pressure. In response to the high arterial pressure transmitted to the thin wall veins, the veins respond by progressive thickening of the muscular layer.

There are two reasons for anastomotic or juxta-anastomotic stenosis. One is trauma due to surgical manipulation and possibly some loss of vasa vasorum in the case of mobilized veins, and the second is neo-intimal hyperplasia caused by turbulent blood flow. The laminar blood flow in the artery becomes turbulent when the high arterial pressure is transmitted to the low-pressure veins because of increased pressure gradient.

The blood flow through the fistula increases quite early after creation. [15] Yerde et. al. showed that the flow through the fistula reaches its maximum flow within 48 hours of creation. Thereon, the flow may reduce if anastomotic stenosis occurs. Wong et al. [16] in their publication showed that not only did the flow through the fistula increase, but the diameter of the outflow vein also increased in all patients after the initial fistula creation during the first two weeks. However, in the subset of patients in whom the fistula did not lead to maturity, the flow through the fistula and the diameter of the outflow vein subsequently decreased. The authors also demonstrated that the size of the vein did not correlate closely to the long-term patency of the fistula. Additionally, Wong et al suggested that the flows measured 24 hours after fistula creation are a more reliable predictor of the patency than the intraoperative flows because of inevitable spasm of the veins due to their handling during surgery. The authors also demonstrated that normal side branches were identified in a majority of the patients, and they were numerous in a minority of the patients.

Robbin et al. describe the ultrasonographic characteristics of the maturing and non-maturing fistulas in their article. [12] They suggest that the outflow veins that do not acquire a diameter of at least 4 mm within 16 weeks of fistula creation and that do not have flow greater than 500 ml/min are less likely to reach maturation. The authors also suggest that an experienced hemodialysis nurse is able to predict the likelihood of a fistula reaching maturity successfully in 80% of cases.

Although the practice of ligation or embolization is quite common among interventional radiologists, interventional nephrologists, and vascular surgeons, there is a dearth of evidence in favor of, or against this practice. Although intuitively and hemodynamically it makes sense to promote higher volume of blood flow through a single outflow vein, one can also argue that leaving the collaterals patent may be beneficial as an alternative hemodialysis access if the main outflow vein becomes unusable at some point. [17] This argument may be valid if there is enough blood flowing through each of the outflow channels to sustain adequate hemodialysis or if there is adequate blood flow through the main hemodialysis outflow vein for adequate hemodialysis despite the presence of competing collaterals. It has been shown that a blood flow of at least 350–500 cc/min is the minimum required for adequate hemodialysis.

Unfortunately, the arterial inflow in many hemodialysis patients is not enough to sustain such levels. Many of these patients are diabetic with severe diabetic vasculopathy compromising arterial inflow. In a study published by Janicki et. al., authors published results in seven patients in whom, they ligated the collateral veins and in whom, the blood flow increased from 260–370 ml/min to over 700 ml/min. [18] Although the study included only seven patients and was not randomized, it does support the notion that ligation or embolization of the collateral veins enhances blood flow through the main inline outflow venous channel and therefore is more likely to produce blood flows required for adequate hemodialysis.

It has also been argued that competing collaterals develop secondary to complete or partial blockage in the main inline outflow vein. [6,7] The authors of this article argue that if the culprit stenosis is adequately treated, embolization or ligation of the competing collateral is never required or even desirable. Turmel-Rodregues et al. claimed that the competing collaterals develop in response to a central stenosis, creating back-pressure forcing development of collaterals. The authors argue that treatment of these veins is neither indicated nor desirable, as angioplasty of the offending lesion will essentially alleviate the problem. Normal venous anatomy, however, indicates that the cephalic as well as basilic veins, prior to creation of fistulas contain side branches. It is not a routine practice of surgeons creating arteriovenous fistulas to debranch the outflow veins. It is therefore evident that a stenotic lesion central to the side branch does not cause these veins; however, if such stenotic lesion is present, it may exaggerate the blood flow through the side branch. In their article, Turmel-Rodrigues et. al. argue that embolization of the collaterals is never indicated, because collateral channels are normal venous branches which become pronounced due to venous hypertension caused central stenosis. Once the stenosis is adequately treated, the collaterals do not fill. [6] The authors also argue that by not adequately dilating the stenosis and instead ligating the collateral, the operator can make the situation worse, leading to fistula thrombosis.

Tessitore et. al. demonstrated a role of prophylactic angioplasty in otherwise functioning virgin native arteriovenous fistulas in a prospective randomized study, demonstrating improved long term patency and reduced morbidity in the patients assigned to the angioplasty arm. [19] The authors showed that preemptive angioplasty of non-hemodynamically significant stenosis can lead to four-fold increase in the patency of the fistula and almost three fold decrease in the likely hood of their failure.

5. Conclusion

In the author's opinion, embolizing and or ligating collateral channels is effective in assisting non-maturating fistula to get to maturation. It is however, difficult to make that claim convincingly without a prospective randomized study. To the best of the authors' knowledge, there has been no prospective randomized study evaluating the effect of ligation or embolization of the collaterals in non-maturing fistulas with or without angioplasty of the stenotic lesion. Such a prospective study is needed to further study the role of collateral vein ligation or embolization in non-maturing hemodialysis fistulas.

Author details

Iftikhar Ahmad*

Minimally Invasive Therapy Specialists, Chicago, IL, USA

References

[1] NKD-K/DOQI "National Kidney Foundation: K/DOQI Clinical Practice Guidelines for Vascular Access." *American journal of Kidney Diseases.* 2001; 37(Suppl 1): S137-S181.

[2] U Bonalumi, D. C., S Rovida et al. "Nine Years experience with end to end arteriovenous fistula at the "anatomical snuffbox" for maintenance hemodialysis." *British Journal of Surgery* 1982; 69: 468-488.

[3] P Kinnaert, P. V., C Toussaint, J Van Geertruyden "Nine years experience with internal arteriovenous fistulas for hemodialysis: A study of some factors infulencing the results." *British Journal of Surgery* 1977; 64: 242-246.

[4] Gerald Beathard, S. S., Marty Shields,"Salvage of the Nonfunctioning arteriovenous fistula." *American journal of Kidney Diseases.*1999; 33: 5.

[5] Luc Turmel-Rodregues, J. P., Harve Rodrigue, Georges Brille, Anne La As E, Dominique Pierre, et al. "Treatment of failed native arteriovenous fistulae for hemodialysis by interventional radilogy." *Kidney International* 2000; 57:1124-1140.

[6] Luc Turmel-Rodrigues, A. M., Beatrice Birmele, Luc Billaux, Naji Ammar, Oliver Gerzard, Serge Hauss, Josette Penglon, "Salvage of immature forearm fistulas for hemodialysis by interventional radiology." *Nephrology Dialysis and Transplantation.* 2001; 16: 2365-2371.

[7] MJ Oliver, R. M., OS Indridason et al. "Comparison of transposed brachiobasilic fistula to upper arm grafts and brachiocephalic fistulas." *Kidney International* 2001; 60: 1532-1539.

[8] BS Dixon, L. N., J Fangman. "Hemodialysis vascular access survival: Upper-arm native arteriovenous fistula." *American journal of Kidney Diseases.* 2002; 39: 92-101.

[9] Gerald Beathard, P. A., Jerry Jackson, Terry Litchfield et al. "Aggressive treatment of early fistula failure." *Kidney International* 2003; 64:

[10] Sheela T. Patel, J. H., Joseph I. Mills, Ariz Tucson. "Failure of arteriovenous fistula maturation: An unintended consequence of exceeding Dialysis Outcome Quality Initiative guidelines for hemodialysis access." *Journal of Vascular Surgery* 2003; 38: 3

[11] Falk, A. "Maintenance and salvage of arteriovenous fistulas." *Journal of Vascular and Interventional Radiology* 2006; 17: 807-813.

[12] ML Robbin, N. C., ME Lockhart, et al. "Hemodialysis arteriovenous fistula maturity: US evaluation." *Radiology* 2002; 225: 59-64.

[13] GA, B. "Physical examination of the dialysis vascular access." *Seminars in Dialysis* 1998; 11: 231-236.

[14] GA, B. "An algorithm for the physical examination of early fistula failure." *Seminars in Dialysis* 2005; 18: 331-335.

[15] MA Yerdel, M. K., KM Yazicioglu, et al. "Effect of hemodynamic variables on surgically created arteriovenous fistula flow." *Nephrology Dialysis and Transplantation.* 1997; 12: 1684-1688.

[16] V. Wong, R. W., J. Taylor, S. Selvakumar, T. V. How, A. Bakran, "Factors associated with early failure of arteriovenous fistulae for hemodialysis access." *European Journal of Vascular and Endovascular Surgery.* 1990; 12:

[17] Ahmad I. Salvage of arteriovenous fistula by angioplasty of collateral veins establishing a new channel. Journal of Vascular Access 2007; 8:123-125.

[18] Krzysztof Janicki, R. P., Anna Bojarska-Szmygin, Janusz Gierynag, Anna Orlowska, Lucyna Janicka. "Chronic dialysis fistula thrombosis treatment by means of endovascular recanalization with surgical exclusion of developed collateral circulation." *Annales Universitatis marie Curie=Sklodowska Lublin-Polonia* 2003; 58: 40.

[19] Nicola Tessitore, G. M., Valeria Bedogna, Giovanni Lipari, Albino Poli, Linda Gammaro, et al. "A prospective controlled trial on effect of percutaneous transluminal angioplasty on funcioning arteriovenous fistulae survival." *Journal of American Society of Nephrology.* 2003; 14:1623.

Section 4

Traumatic Arteriovenous Fistula

Chapter 10

Traumatic Arteriovenous Fistula

Grace Carvajal Mulatti, André Brito Queiroz and
Erasmo Simão da Silva

Additional information is available at the end of the chapter

http://dx.doi.org/10.5772/56368

1. Introduction

Vascular injuries caused by civilian or war trauma represent a surgical challenge. These lesions are potentially lethal and can cause death at the scene. One of the most fascinating and misdiagnosed complications of vascular injuries is the arteriovenous fistula (AVF), which results from a direct communication between an artery and a vein. They are usually secondary to penetrating trauma and occasionally may be diagnosed many years after the injury.

2. Historic data

Knowledge and experience on vascular trauma was obtained especially in wartime. In 1757 William Hunter has described the physiopathology associated with an AVF and since then the management of these clinical problem has challenged many surgeons.

In addition to case reports of the 19th Century, there have been many published series resulting from wartime experience throughout the 20th Century. Much of the experience acquired from treating and diagnosing AVF comes from the II World War and the Korean and Vietnam Wars. In the Korean conflict as many as 215 fistulas and aneurysms have been described. Cumulative, fistulas and false aneurysms may account for 7 % of the casualties in Vietnam. At that time, diagnosis was established by physical examination with palpation and auscultation, and confirmed by arteriography.

Most cases of arteriovenous fistulas and pseudoaneurysms were treated conservatively in wartime, and operated only later.

Most recently, experience has been obtained from the Iraq and Afghanistan wars. Treatment has evolved over the past decades thanks to the endovascular techniques, however early diagnosing still seems to be a challenge. Even in recent studies arteriovenous fistulas are frequently occult findings and are diagnosed only when an arteriogram is performed.

3. Etiology

Traumatic AVFs are usually caused by penetrating trauma, accounting for as many as 90 % of cases. Blunt trauma is rarely the cause and it is responsible for the other 10 %. Gunshot wounds are the most frequent ones, but stab wounds and iatrogenic lesions may also account for traumatic AVFs.

Most of the military trauma injuries affect the extremities. On the other hand extremities and abdominal injuries are equally distributed in the civilian population.

Traumatic AVFs often result from a cold weapon or a small-caliber bullet, as high-velocity lesions are usually cause of hemorrhage and potentially hemodynamic shock (Fig 1 and 2).

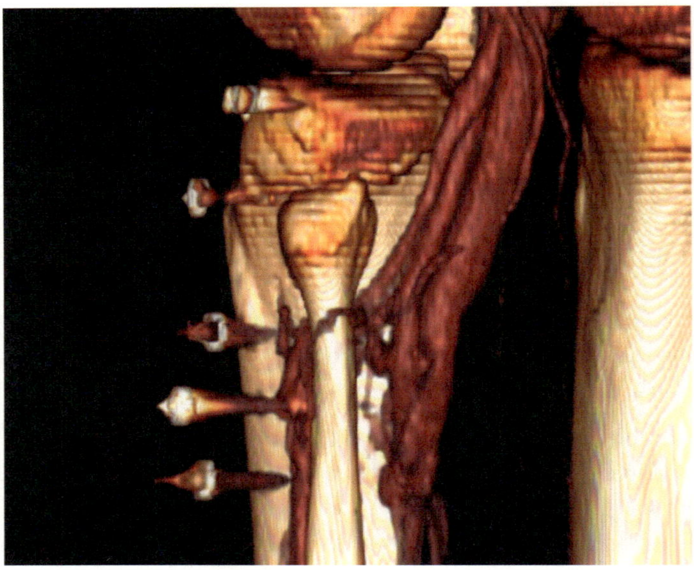

Figure 1. Three-dimensional computed tomography (CT) reconstruction shows an AVF involving below the the knee vessels and multiple bullet shrapnel near the lesion.

When it comes from iatrogenic lesions, the most frequent are the ones caused by percutaneous interventions such as renal biopsies, cardiac catheterization and orthopedic procedures. Therapeutic procedures and their complexity increase the risk. Following cardiac catheterization the femoral AVF is the most common. Nonetheless it has also been reported carotid or subclavian AVFs following placement of a central venous catheters.

http://dx.doi.org/10.5772/56368

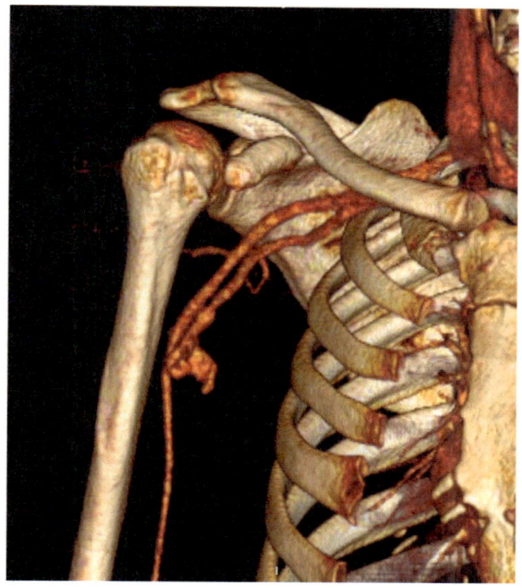

Figure 2. Three dimensional CT reconstruction shows a brachial AVF associated with a pseudoaneurysm after a stab wound in the arm.

Carotid-cavernous fistulae (CCF) are usually traumatic and potentially lethal. Mechanisms include fractures to the base of the skull, penetrating wounds and even more rarely rupture of preexisting aneurysms.

4. Clinical signs

Post-traumatic AVF is an unusual disease with a wide variability of presentations. They are often asymptomatic, but when significant can cause rapid shunting with return of oxygenated blood to the right heart. Clinical signs may be detected from a few hours to many years after the injury and may vary according to the location and diameter of the affected vessels.

The clinical diagnosis of a traumatic AVF is based on a history of trauma and meticulous physical examination. Physical examination with palpation and auscultation may reveal thrills, murmurs, bruits and a pulsatile mass. Distal pulses may be palpable, but the AVF can shunt away blood from the extremity and cause symptoms of distal ischemia.

The Nicoladoni-Israel-Branham's sign may be present: the manual compression of the fistula or the artery proximal to the fistula causes a decrease in the heart rate. This maneuver produces an increase in peripheral vascular resistance and afterload. The response to the increased afterload is a reflex bradycardia.

In a trauma scenario bone fractures or neurologic deficits can raise the suspicion of a vascular injury, especially when the physical examination is not remarkable.

Chronic fistulas are even more rare, and large flow AVFs can present with symptoms of high output congestive heart failure, edema and cardiomegaly. Those more prompt to develop a delayed presentation are young trauma victims.

Aneurysmal degeneration of the involved arterial and venous segments may also occur due to structural changes secondary to hemodynamic stress (Fig 3). Fistulas affecting the extremities may lead to signs of venous hypertension, varicosities, pain and limb overgrowth. Pulsatile varicose veins can draw attention to the pathology lying underneath (Fig 4 and 5).

As regard to CCF, clinical signs include pulsatile exophthalmos, eyeball redness, bruit, diplopia, ptosis, visual disturbances, and loss of visual acuity. During physical examination it has been observed that the bruit shall disappear should the examiner occlude the ICA by digital compression.

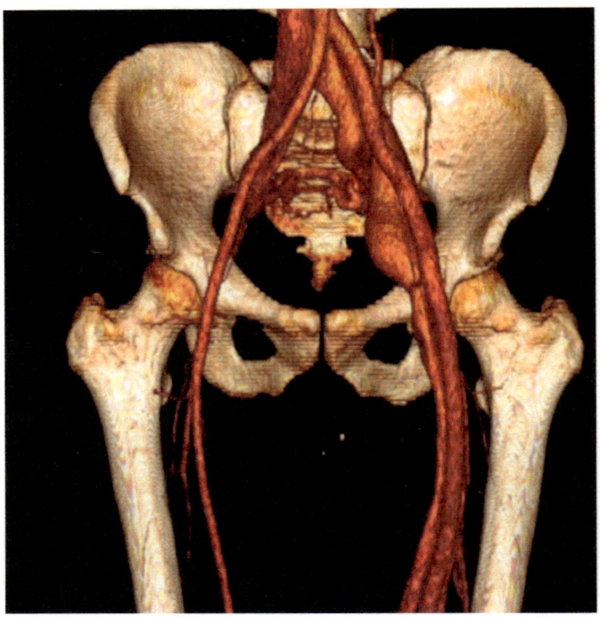

Figure 3. Three-dimensional CT reconstruction shows aneurysmal degeneration of iliac and femoral arteries and veins secondary to an AVF involving below the knee vessels.

According to literature, the most frequent locations are the femoral and popliteal vessels. Other sites include aorto-caval, iliac, carotid-jugular and renal fistulas.

The differential diagnosis must include pseudoaneurysm, true aneurysm, arteriovenous malformation, cyst, abscess and hematoma. One must remember that nonvascular lesions may appear pulsatile due to transmitted pulsation from adjacent arteries.

http://dx.doi.org/10.5772/56368

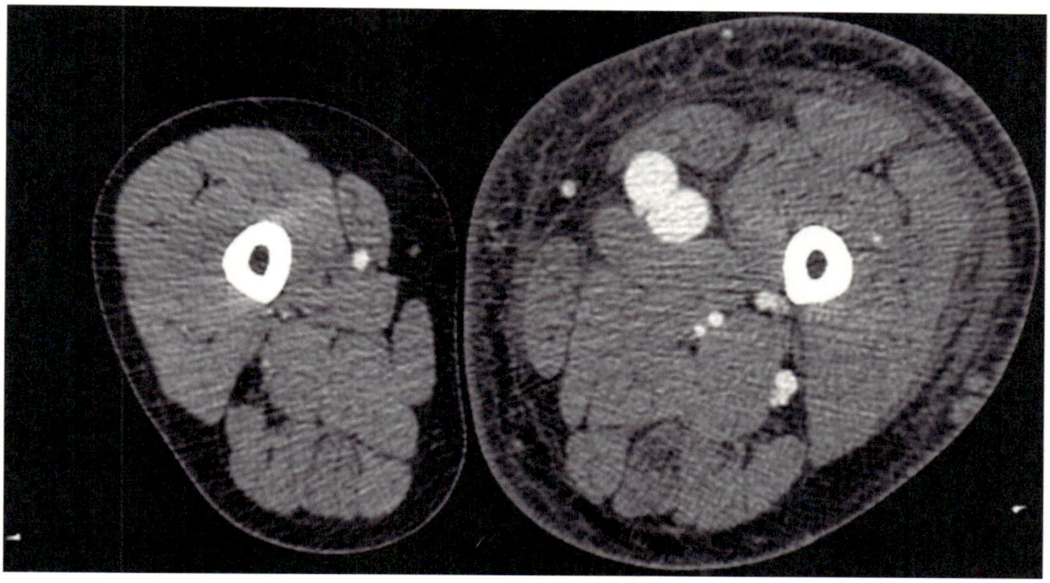

Figure 4. Contrast-enhanced CT demonstrates an AVF between femoral artery and vein, secondary to a gunshot wound 15 years earlier, with left lower limb overgrowth and venous hypertension.

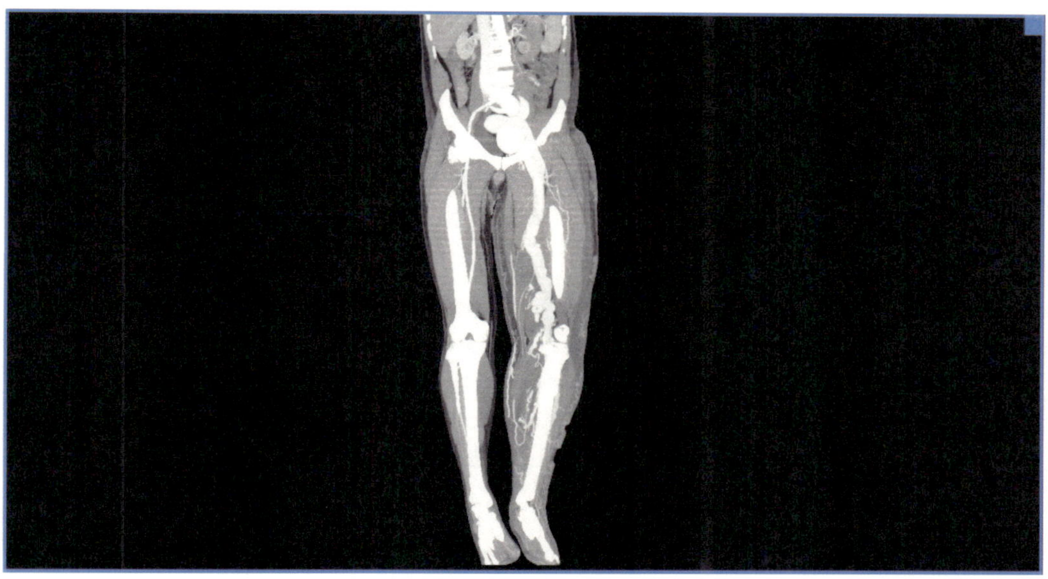

Figure 5. The same patient of figure 4, computed tomography in coronal view demonstrates left lower limb overgrowth and dilated iliac and femoral vessels.

5. Diagnostic imaging

Diagnosis is usually difficult and greatly dependent on imaging studies. Arteriography was the main exam in the 1960 and 1970s and still plays an important role in diagnosing AVF. However, nowadays the computed tomography (CT) angiography, magnetic resonance imaging (MRI) and color Doppler have been playing an important role in the diagnosis of this pathology.

Arteriography is still the gold standard exam for diagnosing vascular traumas, including traumatic AVFs. Catheter based angiography is a dynamic study and can, in most cases accurately demonstrates the arteries filling the fistula and the exact point of the arteriovenous communication. The major disadvantages of conventional arteriography are the cost of the procedure, the delay that occurs before arteriography, and the need for a specialized team comprising a physician, angiography technologist, and nurse. Besides being an invasive exam that requires an arterial access it can result in a number of different complications.

Computed tomographic angiography is a reliable and convenient imaging modality for diagnosing AVF after blunt and penetrating trauma. It is a noninvasive modality that could replace conventional arteriography as the initial diagnostic study for arterial injuries after trauma, even when the suspected diagnosis is an AVF. The technique requires scanning with multidetector helical CT after rapid intravenous injection of iodinated contrast material. This is a noninvasive, accurate, and easily accessible diagnostic imaging test acquired by a single trained technologist.

In recent years CT is increasingly available in the emergency setting. The development of helical CT scanners with a multi-detector row configuration and three-dimensional postprocessing has further encouraged the use of CT angiography in the evaluation of a suspected vascular injury. High quality axial images and reformatted angiography exams can be obtained in a shorter time than with other modalities and with a lesser complication rate than catheter angiography.

In some cases metallic streak artifact, motion artifact, and inadequate arterial opacification may render a CT angiogram nondiagnostic. Streak artifacts are the major limiting factor of CT angiography to demonstrate AVFs after penetrating missile injuries. The deposited metallic fragments may create streak artifacts that obscure the arteries, commonly at the exact location where the AVF is likely to occur (Fig. 6). In these cases, angiography is necessary for optimal assessment.

Contrast-enhanced CT has also an important role in surgical planning because it can reveal where the lesion is, its extension, and its relation to adjacent structures, mainly in the abdominal or thoracic cavities. It is also important for endovascular treatment planning allowing precise measurements of the diameters and length of involved vessels. Computed tomography and MRI typically show early contrast filling in the vein during the arterial phase (Fig. 7).

http://dx.doi.org/10.5772/56368

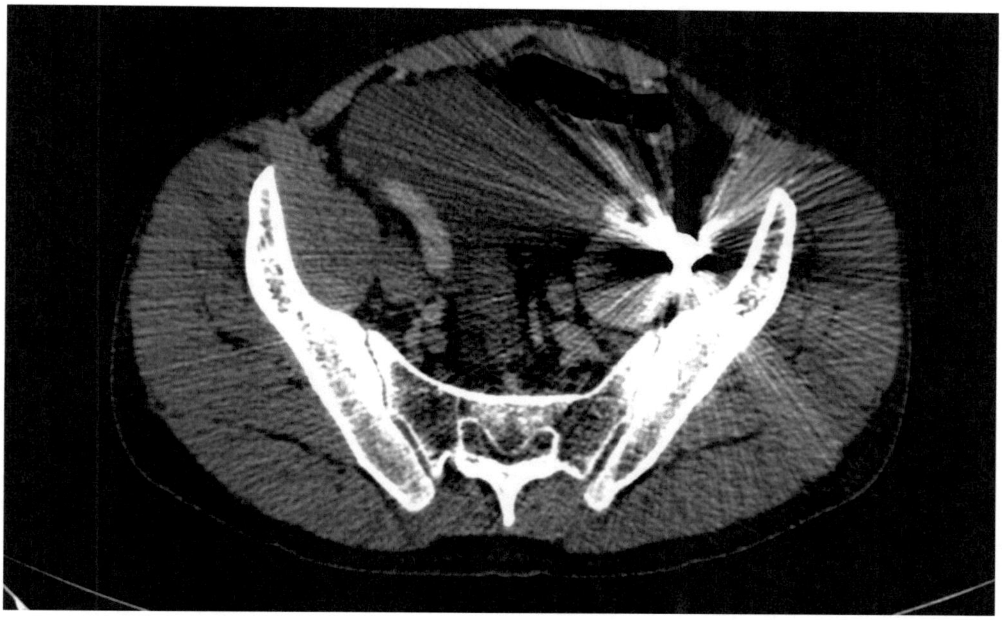

Figure 6. Computed tomography in a patient who sustained an iliac AVF with bullet fragments obscuring the vessels near the arteriovenous communication

Angiography and CT share the same complications rates related to the use of iodinated contrast, like allergic reactions and renal function impairment and requires also the use of radiation for execution.

Some authors have also proposed MRI for assessment of vascular injuries including traumatic AVF, but it may be limited for depiction of concurrent osseous injuries. Furthermore, MR is not well suited for some patients with impacted metallic fragments and acutely injured ones requiring life support devices as they may be not compatible with the magnet.

In chronic AVF both the artery and the vein dilate and elongate in response to the greater blood flow and shear stress, but the vein dilates more and becomes "arterialized". Findings include a pseudoaneurysm, large venous aneurysms, proximal dilation of the artery or hematoma of the vessel wall (Fig. 7).

In the setting of a suspected AVF, not confirmed by physical findings, the color doppler, a simple non-invasive method can usually clear out the diagnosis. Gray-scale ultrasound imaging is not helpful in the evaluation of acute AVF, although may be important in chronic AVF when the high flow state has caused dilatation of the vein and artery. Color doppler imaging is usually diagnostic. Tissue vibrations caused by turbulent flow are the most notable color Doppler finding. Also, the exact spot of the arteriovenous communication can sometimes be identified. The Doppler waveform in the feeding artery shows a low resistance pattern with increased diastolic flow. The jet of arterial flow entering the vein can cause a marked flow disturbance and chaotic waveform or an arterial waveform is present in more severe cases (Fig 8, 9).

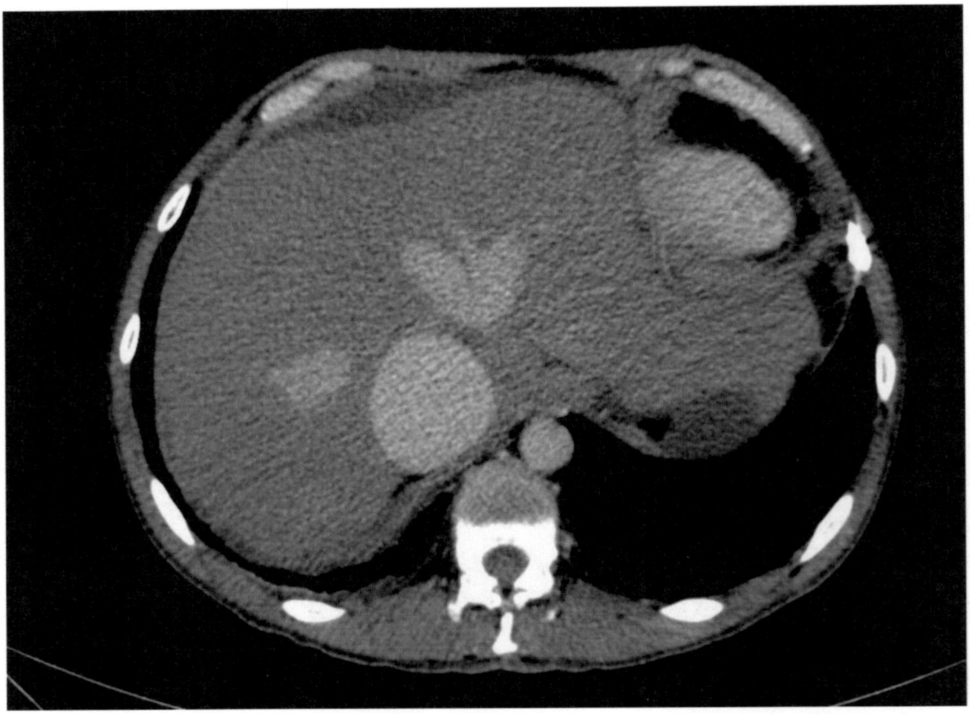

Figure 7. Contrast-enhanced CT shows dilated inferior vena cava with the same contrast opacification of the aorta in the arterial phase in a patient with iliac AVF.

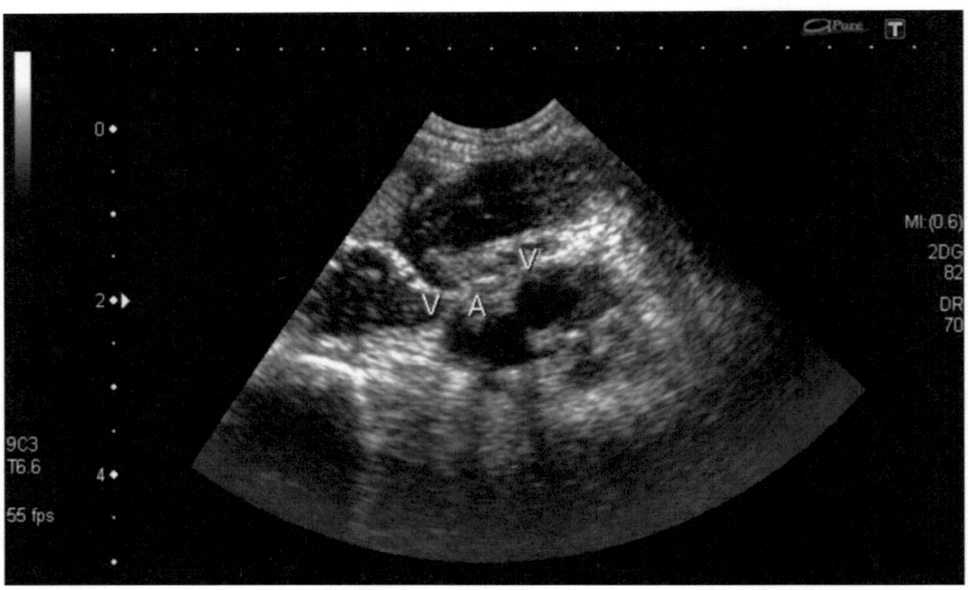

Figure 8. Ultrasound demonstrates the arteriovenous communication in a brachial AVF secondary to a stab wound.

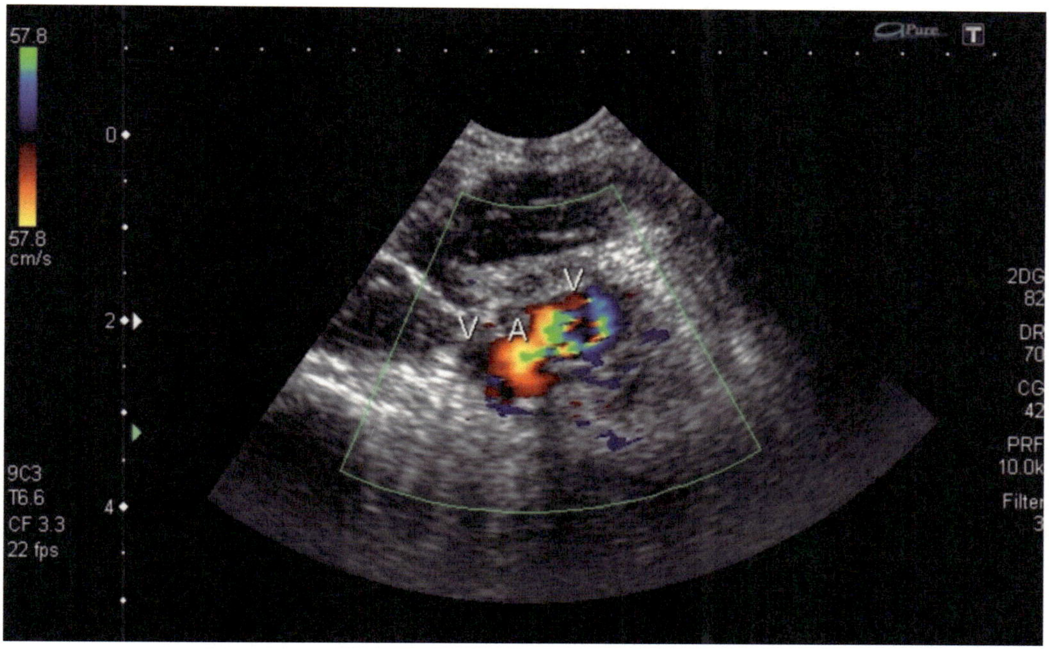

Figure 9. Color Doppler shows the communication between the brachial artery and vein with marked flow disturbance in the same patient of figure 2.

All imaging studies used in the diagnosis of arterial or venous diseases may play a role in traumatic AVF diagnosing. Nowadays color doppler and CT angiography are the usual exams, and the catheter based angiography is performed only for the more complex cases and as confirmatory exam or when it is necessary for planning the endovascular treatment.

6. Treatment

Early recognition and prompt repair may lead to a significant decrease in the number of complications such as congestive heart failure or venous hypertension of the limb. AVFs do not resolve spontaneously in the majority cases. The aim of the treatment is the closure of the AVF, with preservation of patency of the main vessels.

Surgical repair using traditional surgical techniques is feasible. However, an open approach for many of these lesions may be fraught with peril owing to grossly distorted and edematous tissue planes. Arterial and venous repair with the saphenous vein or prosthetic graft were largely used in the war series and are still used nowadays. Venous ligation can be used depending on its diameter, quadruple ligation-excision and complex reconstructions may be used. However, late presentation of AVF is prone to significant intraoperative bleeding due to the complex venous anatomy encountered during surgical dissection and repair. Associated morbidities can include limb ischemia, gangrene, limb loss, Vena Cava thrombosis, pulmonary embolus, venous stasis, and uncontrollable bleeding.

In an effort to avoid the morbidity and mortality associated with an open approach for traumatic AVFs, the focus has shifted to endovascular techniques. The main advantage of endovascular approach is that the system can be inserted through a remote access site, obviating the need for extensive surgical exposure. Endovascular repair can include the use of covered stents and coil embolization, depending on the location and diameter of the involved vessels. In some cases open surgical repair has prohibitive morbidity and mortality, and a minimal invasive technique has emerged as an effective treatment alternative. Recognized advantages of endovascular repair for traumatic AVF compared with open repair include diminished pain, decreased disability and rapid recovery. The first recorded repair of an AVF using an endovascular approach was in 1992 by Parodi when a covered stent was deployed to treat a traumatic AVF in subclavian vessels.

The goal of endovascular therapy is the selective elimination of the vascular lesion, with the preservation of normal patency of the essential vessels. Endovascular therapy using covered stents and coils are both feasible and safe for treating traumatic AVF. Of these endovascular methods, stent-graft placement can be used to exclude the fistula from circulation and preserve the parent artery and vein. Embolization with coils may be used in selective cases, when nonessential vessels are responsible for the arteriovenous communication, and both procedures may be associated. Complications during covered stent placement are due to dissection or rupture and embolization of the devices causing ischemic complications.

Subacute thrombosis and intimal hyperplasia leading to in-stent stenosis or vessel occlusion are other complications associated with covered stents. The long-term patency of these devices is unknown. Some authors consider that balloon-expandable covered stents like Advanta V12 (Atrium, USA) are better when accurate deployment is required. We believe that newer self-expanding devices, such as Fluency (Bard, USA) and Viabahn (Gore, USA), which are stent

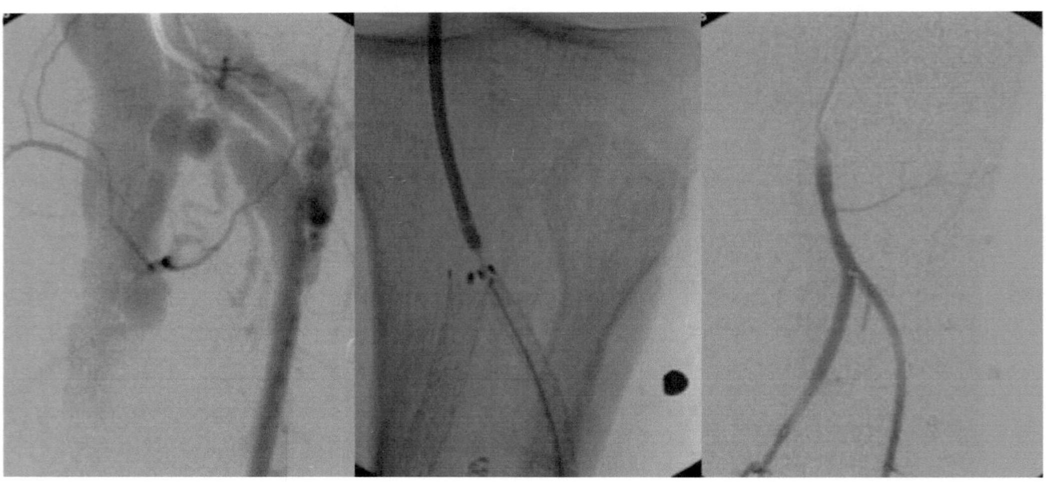

Figure 10. Sequential figures show catheter-based angiography demonstrating AVF in tibial anterior and posterior vessels, subsequent self-expanding covered stents deployment and final arteriography demonstrating closure of the arteriovenous communication.

grafts composed of nitinol stents covered with polytetrafluoroethylene, are more flexible, conform more easily to the vessel walls, and the polytetrafluoroethylene covering is less thrombogenic. Therefore, we thought that these devices appear to be more suitable. When chronic AVF presents with very enlarged vessels the use of endografts primarily designed for aortic and iliac diseases may be used in aorto-iliac and other vessels (Fig. 10,11, 12).

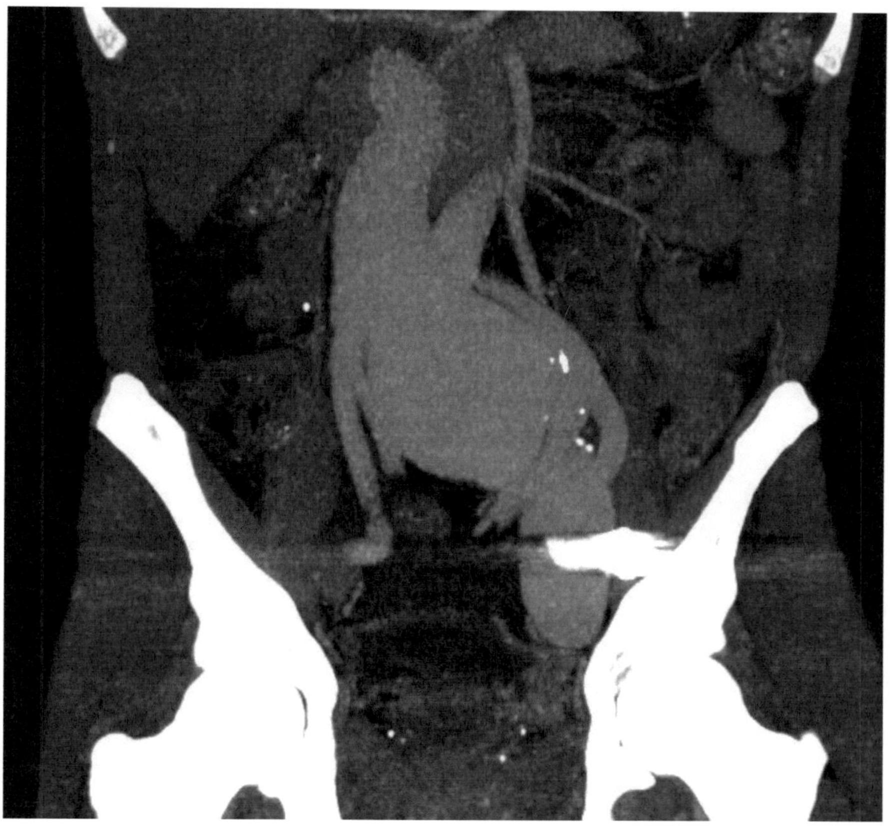

Figure 11. Computed tomography in coronal view show an iliac AVF dilated iliac veins and inferior vena cava, with the same contrast opacification.

Due to the reduced venous flow following AVF closure, venous thrombosis can occur especially when venous aneurysms are present, carrying out complications like pulmonary embolism. In this situation systemic anticoagulation is recommended for at least six months after the AVF treatment. Inferior vena cava filters may have significant importance in some cases, however attention to the diameter of these veins is essential to prevent migration of the filters.

Neuroradiologists or interventional radiologists usually carry out treatment of CCFs with innumerous endovascular possibilities, such as coil embolization, double balloon occlusion technique or occlusion of the ICA by use of detachable balloon, the last being the gold standard.

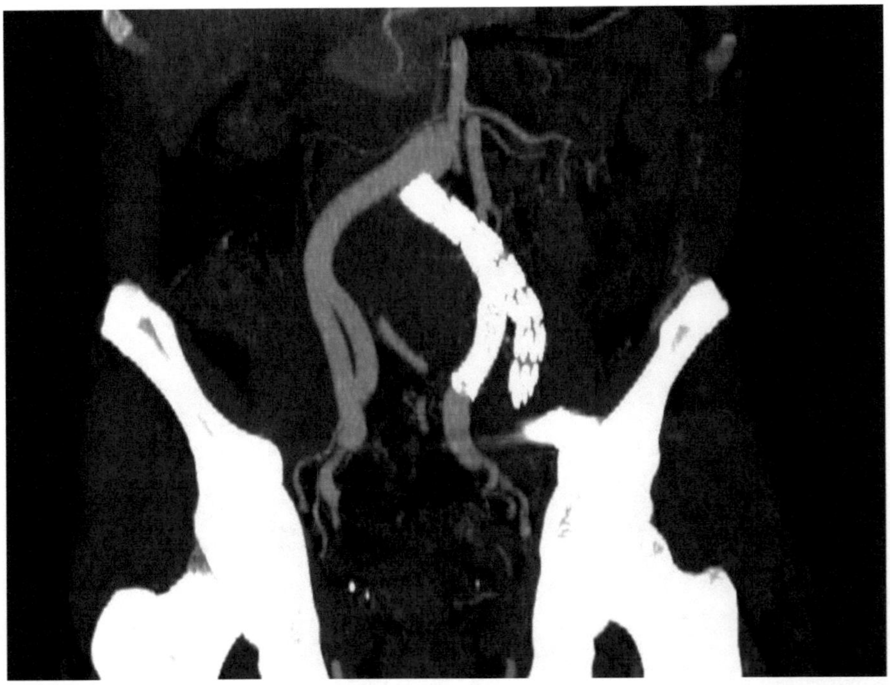

Figure 12. Computed tomography in coronal view of the same patient in figure 10 after endovascular treatment with covered devices demonstrates no venous opacification and pervious iliac arteries.

Author details

Grace Carvajal Mulatti, André Brito Queiroz and Erasmo Simão da Silva

Vascular and Endovascular Surgery Division, São Paulo University Medical School, São Paulo-SP, Brazil

References

[1] Anderson, C. A, & Strumpf, R. K. Dietricht EB: Endovascular management of a large post-traumatic iliac arteriovenous fistula: Utilization of a septal occlusion device. J Vasc Surg (2008). , 48, 1597-9.

[2] Creech, O, & Gantt, J. Wren H: Traumatic Arteriovenous Fistula at Unusual Sites. Ann Surg. (1965). June; , 161(6), 908-920.

[3] Davison, B. D, & Polak, J. F. Arterial injuries: a sonographic approach. Radiol Clin North Am. (2004). Mar;, 42(2), 383-96.

[4] DuBose JRecinos G, Teixeira PG, Inaba K, Demetriades D. Endovascular stenting for the treatment of traumatic internal carotid injuries: expanding experience. J Trauma. (2008). Dec;, 65(6), 1561-6.

[5] Fattahi, T. T, Brandt, T, Jenkins, W. S, & Steinberg, B. Traumatic Carotid-Cavernous Fistula: Pathophysiology and Treatment. J Craniof Surg. (2003). Mar;, 14(2), 240-6.

[6] Faure, E, Canaud, L, Marty-ané, C, & Alric, P. Endovascular repair of a left common carotid pseudoaneurysm associated with a jugular-carotid fistula after gunshot wound to the neck. Ann Vasc Surg. (2012). Nov;26(8):1129.e, 13-6.

[7] Faure, E, Canaud, L, & Marty-ané, C. Alric P: endovascular Repair of a Left Common Carotid Pseudoaneurysm Associated With a Jugular-Carotid Fistula After Gunshot Wound to the Neck. Ann Surg, (2012). ee16., 13-1129.

[8] Feliciano, D. V, Bitondo, C. G, Mattox, K. L, et al. Civilian trauma in the 1980's. A 1-year experience with 456 vascular and cardiac injuries. Ann Surg (1984). , 199, 717-723.

[9] Fox, C. J, Gillespie, D. L, & Donnell, O. SD, et al: Contemporary management of wartime vascular trauma. J Vasc Surg (2005). , 41, 638-644.

[10] Huang, W, Villavicencio, J. L, & Rich, N. M. Delayed treatment and late complications of a traumatic arteriovenous fistula. J Vasc Surg. (2005). Apr;, 41(4), 715-7.

[11] Hughes CW: Arterial repair during the Korean WarAnn Surg (1958). , 147, 555-561.

[12] Nagpal, K, Ahmed, K, & Cuschieri, R. J. Diagnosis and management of acute traumatic arteriovenous fistula. Int J Angiol (2008). , 17(4), 214-216.

[13] Khoury, G, Sfeir, R, Nabbout, G, Jabbour-khoury, S, & Fahl, M. Traumatic arteriovenous fistulae: "the Lebanese war experience". Eur J Vasc Surg. (1994). Mar;, 8(2), 171-3.

[14] Kim, J. W, Kim, S. J, & Kim, M. R. Traumatic carotid-cavernous sinus fistula accompanying abducens nerve (VI) palsy in blowout fractures: missed diagnosis of "white-eyed shunt". Int J Oral Maxillofac Surg. (2013). Apr;, 42(4), 470-3.

[15] Kollmeyer, K. R, Hunt, J. L, Ellman, B. A, & Fry, W. J. Acute and chronic traumatic arteriovenous fistulae in civilians. Arch Surg (1981). , 116, 697-702.

[16] Kuhlencordt, P. J, Linsenmeyer, U, Rademacher, A, et al. Large external iliac vein aneurysm in a patient with a post-traumatic femoral arteriovenous fistula. J Vasc Surg (2008). , 47, 205-8.

[17] Miller-thomas, M. M, West, O. C, & Cohen, A. M. Diagnosing traumatic arterial injury in the extremities with CT angiography: pearls and pitfalls. Radiographics. (2005). Oct;25 Suppl 1:S, 133-42.

[18] Parodi, J, & Barone, H. Transluminal treatment of abdominal aortic aneurysms and peripheral arteriovenous fistulas. Presented at the 19th Annual Montefiore Medical

Center Symposium on Current Critical Problems and New Techniques in Vascular Surgery, New York, NY, Nov 21, (1992).

[19] Queiroz, A. B, Mulatti, G. C, Aun, R, et al. Endovascular repair of a traumatic arteriovenous fistula involving the iliac bifurcation using an iliac branch device. J Vasc Surg. (2012). May;, 55(5), 1474-6.

[20] Hewitt, R L. and D J Collins Acute arteriovenous fistulas in war injuries. Ann Surg. (1969). March; , 169(3), 447-449.

[21] Spencer, T. A, Smyth, S. H, Wittich, G, et al. Delayed presentation of traumatic aortocaval fistula: A report of two cases and a review of the associated compensatory hemodynamic and structural changes. J Vasc Surg (2006). , 43, 836-40.

[22] Drapanas, T, Hewitt, R L, Weichert, R F, & Rd, A. D Smith Civilian vascular injuries: a critical appraisal of three decades of management. Ann Surg. (1970). September; , 172(3), 351-360.

[23] Takenoshita, Y, Hasuoz, K, Matsushima, T, & Oka, M. Carotid-Cavernous Sinus Fistula Accompanying Facial Trauma: Report of a Case with a Review of the Literature. J Cranio-Max Fac Surg. (1990). , 18, 41-5.

[24] Yu, P. T, Rice-townsend, S, Naheedy, J, Almodavar, H, & Mooney, D. P. Delayed presentation of traumatic infrapopliteal arteriovenous fistula and pseudoaneursym in a year-old boy managed by coil embolization. J Pediatr Surg. (2012). Feb;47(2):e7-10., 10.

Chapter 11

Traumatic Middle Meningeal Artery and Fistula Formation with the Cavernous Sinus and a Review of the Literature on Endovascular Management of Traumatic Carotid Cavernous Fistulas

Xianli Lv, Youxiang Li and Chuhan Jiang

Additional information is available at the end of the chapter

http://dx.doi.org/10.5772/56352

1. Introduction

Traumatic carotid-cavernous fistula of Barrow Type C is uncommon complication of head trauma[Table1].[1-8] This vascular lesion might be missed unless it exhibits clinical manifestations or are incidentally discovered during radiological examination such as magnetic resonance imaging or conventional angiography.[1-8] Here we present a case of traumatic middle meningeal artery, which subsequently established a fistula with the cavernous sinus. We also discuss the methods used for treatment of traumatic carotid cavernous fistulas[TCCFs].

Type	Description
A	Supply from the internal carotid artery
B	Supply from the dural branches of internal carotid artery
C	Supply from the dural branches of external carotid artery
D	Combined forms

Table 1. Barrow types of CCF.

2. Case report

A 22-year-old man suffered blunt head trauma in a basket-ball game and was admitted to a local hospital. Physical examination at the time of administration showed normal. Skull radiographs showed no skull fracture. He was managed conservatively. One month later, intracranial bruits developed subsequently demonstrated intracranial bruits developed and subsequently demonstrated blurred vision, left exophthalmos, diplopia and blepharoptosis. Magnetic resonance vision, left exophthalmos, diplopia and blepharoptosis. Magnetic resonance imaging [MRI] revealed the dilated left superior ophthalmic vein [Fig.1]. Cerebral angiography demonstrated the fistula was located exactly at the foramen spinosum, and drained into the ipsilateral cavernous sinus through a dural sinus on the floor of middle cranial fossa[Fig.2,3]. There was also a dilated cortical vein draining into the superior sagittal sinus.

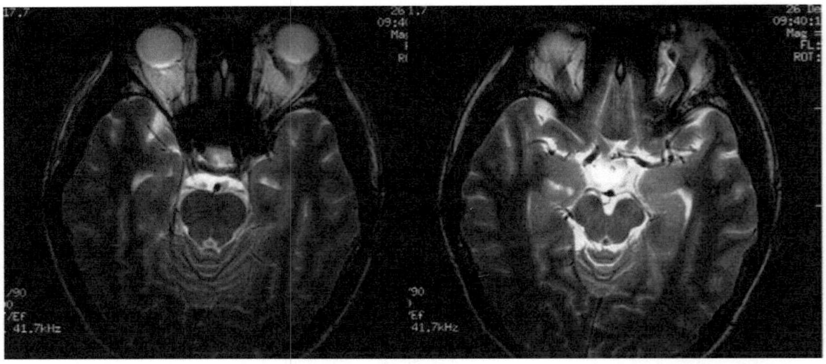

Figure 1. Axial T2-weighted magnetic resonance image showed the left dilated ophthalmic vein.

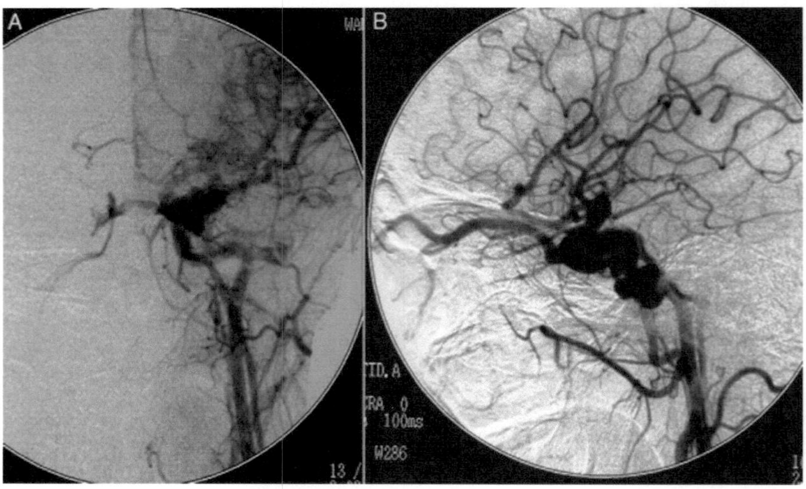

Figure 2. Angiograms of left common carotid artery, frontal[A] and lateral[B], demonstrated, a carotid-cavernous -cavernous fistula like Barrow Type A.

http://dx.doi.org/10.5772/56352

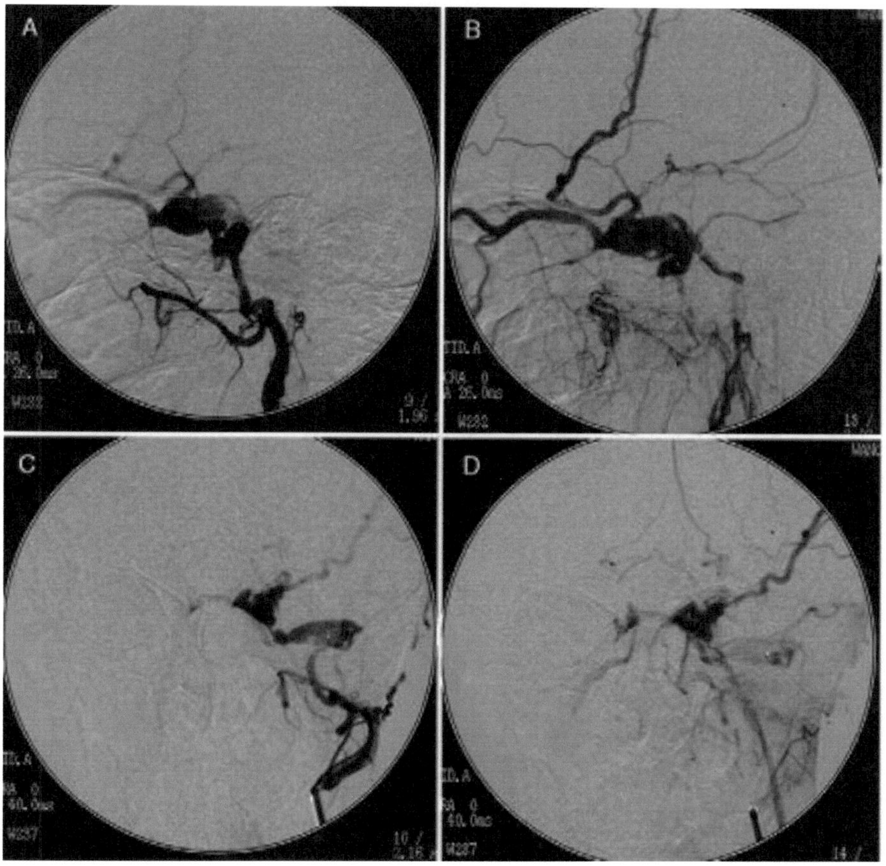

Figure 3. Angiorams of the left external carotid artery injection, lateral projection, arterial phase[A] and late arterial phase[B], anteroposterior projection, arterial phase[C] and late arterial phase[D], demonstrated the fistuta fed by by the dilated left middle meningeal artery and drained into the left superior ophthalmic vein and a cortical vein.

2.1. Intervention

The procedure was performed with an 8-F guiding catheter [Cordis, USA] catheterized into the left external carotid artery and 3000 U heparin were administered intravenously. Then a Magic-BD microcatheter caring a 3# detachable balloon [Balt, Montmorency, France] was advanced through the guiding catheter up to the fistula via the dilated left middle meningeal artery. An immediate obliteration of the DAVF was achieved after the balloon was inflated with 0.3ml contrast injection [Fig.4,5]. The procedure was ended.

2.2. Postprocedure course

The postprocedure course was uneventful. The patient was discharged home on the postprocedure day2 without any neurologic abnormalities. One month clinical follow-up demonstrated no intracranial bruits.

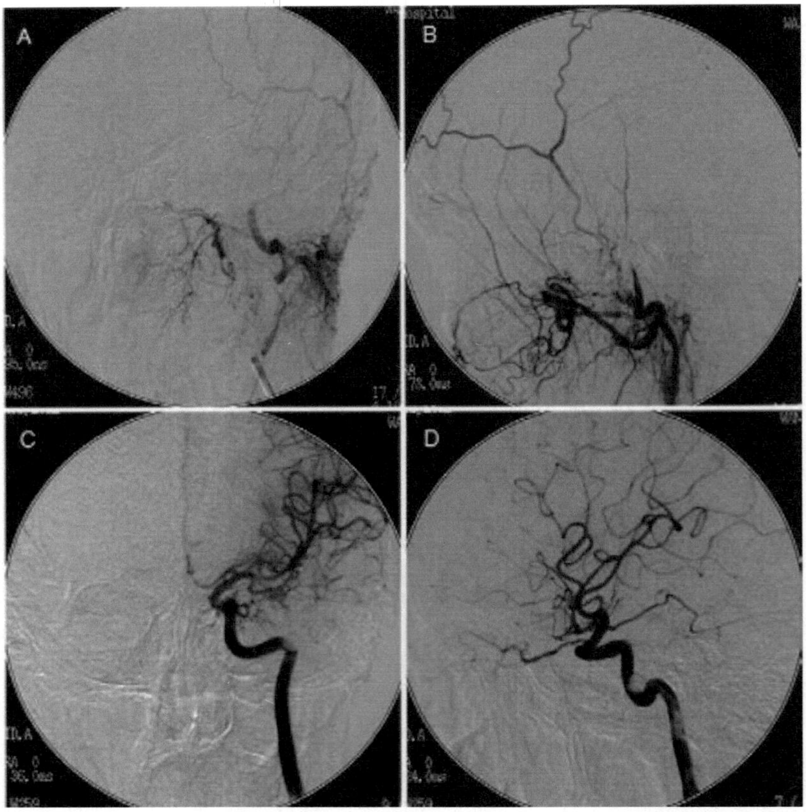

Figure 4. Postembolization angiogram, left external carotid injection, frontal[A] and lateral[B] and left internal carotid injection, frontal[C] and lateral[D], demonstrated immediate obliteration of the fistula.

3. Discussion

The present case demonstrated an unusual DAVF caused by laceration of the meningeal artery and opening of a venous lake adjacent to the cavernous sinus. Many cases of middle meningeal fistula in association with head trauma were reported.[1-12] However, we are not aware of a reported case treated by detachable balloon and without skull fracture. In the present case, one month passed between head injury and the appearance of intracranial bruits. The case can be considered one of chronic DAVF based on this relatively asymptomatic interval. A delayed onset of symptoms is mainly attributable to disruption of dural venous drainage and increased intracavernous pressure.[1-3,5,8] Neurosurgeons should be aware of this possibility that DAVF in the middle meningeal artery in patients without skull fracture. In our case, initially the common carotid angiography was performed [Fig.2] and the lesion was misdiagnosed as Barrow Type A. However, the selective external carotid angiograms demonstrated a DAVF of Barrow Type C in the middle cranial fossa. Endovascular embolization is the treatment choice of the DAVF of the middle meningeal artery, and has some advantages over surgical treatment.[1,3-5,9] Embolic materials should be selected

http://dx.doi.org/10.5772/56352

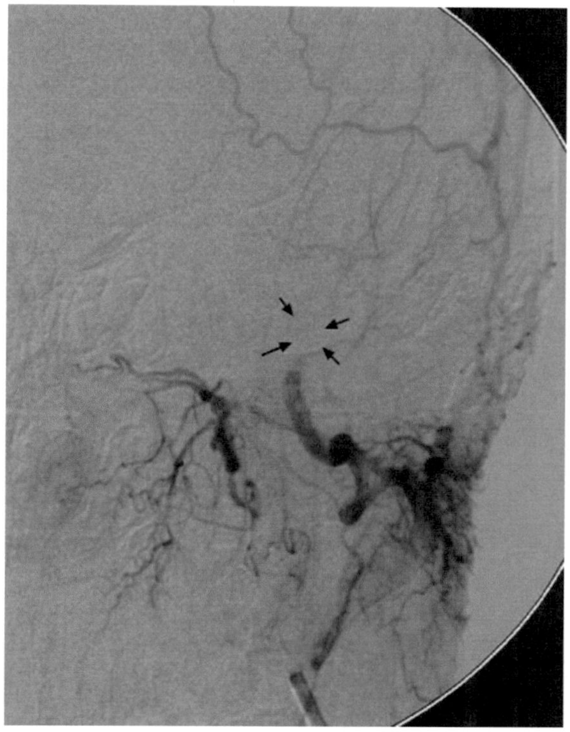

Figure 5. Angiogram showed the dilated detachable balloon obliterating the fistula[Arrow heads].

carefully depending on the type and size of the lesions to prevent complications and recanalization.[1,3-5,9] In our cases, we used detachable balloon to treat the DAVF, which resulted in successful embolization.

4. Review of endovascular management of traumatic carotid-cavernous fistulas

Ever since the use of balloons for the treatment of TCCFs was described by Debrun et al[13] and Serbinenko,[14] transarterial balloon embolization has been the criterion standard treatment for most patients with TCCF. Higashida et al. [15] reported preservation of the parent artery in 88% of patients with TCCFs treated by using detachable balloons; other authors have described a need for parent artery occlusion in as many as 20% of cases[16,17].

Technical difficulties are not uncommon in balloon embolization and are related to the size of the fistula and the cavernous sinus [18]. The fistula should be smaller than an inflated balloon but large enough to allow passage of a deflated or partially inflated balloon, and the CS should be large enough to accommodate an inflated balloon or balloons. Complications related to detachable balloon embolization of TCCFs are not uncommon and include venous stasis, orbital congestion, cerebral ischemia [3%], cerebral infarction [4%], and permanent neurologic damage [3%][19]. Third and sixth nerve palsy after balloon embolization has also been observed. Debrun et al.[20] reported a 20% incidence of transient oculomotor nerve palsy, which is usually combined to sixth cranial nerve dysfunction.

Failure often occurs when the fistula orifice is too small to allow entry or when a large fistula is combined with a small CS, allowing retraction of the inflated balloon into the ICA[21]. For TCCFs that are not successfully treated by using a detachable balloon, transarterial GDC embolization is an alternative treatment. In 1992, Guglielmi et al.[22] successfully treated TCCFs by transvenous GDC embolization, and there have been several subsequent reports of transarterial GDC embolization of TCCFs with favorable results[23-25]. The advantages of using GDCs are the ability to control their placement and easy retrieval and repositioning or exchange if necessary. It is also technically easier to guide a microcatheter and microguidewire combination through a small fistula than a balloon. Transarterial NBCA or ONYX embolization of TCCFs has been reported to be an efficient treatment for TCCFs when a trans arterial detachable balloon or GDC fails to seal the fistula; this procedure has the advantage of being relatively easy to deliver through a microcatheter, producing rapid induction of thrombosis and permanent occlusion after polymerization or solidification [26-28].

An investigation described that the risk of oculomotor nerve deficit was significantly higher when using a detachable balloon than a GDC for the treatment of TCCF [29]. A possible reason for the occurrence of oculomotor palsy may be over inflation or migration of the balloon, leading to direct compression of the cranial nerves. In contrast, a GDC is very pliable and adapts to the shape of the CS without exerting a significant mass effect on the cranial nerves [22].

Many surgical methods for simple neck ipsilateral carotid artery ligation method, now largely abandoned. Currently, the mainstay of treatment for TCCF is endovascular therapy. This may be transarterial or transvenous.[30] Occasionally, more direct approaches, such as direct transorbital puncture of the cavernous sinus or cannulation of the draining superior orbital vein are used when conventional approaches are not possible.[31,32] TCCF may be treated by occlusion of the affected cavernous sinus [coils, balloon, NBCA or ONYX], or by reconstruction of the damaged internal carotid artery [stent, coils, NBCA or ONYX].

5. Conclusion

The middle meningeal fistula can be presented due to head trauma, even there is no skull fracture. Selective external carotid angiogram is necessary for correct diagnosis and endovascular embolization is an effective way. Endovascular embolization of TCCFs using detachable balloons, coils with or without NBCA or ONYX combination was considered to be a feasible, effective, and safe method for the treatment.

http://dx.doi.org/10.5772/56352

Author details

Xianli Lv, Youxiang Li and Chuhan Jiang

Beijing Neurosurgical Institute and Beijing Tiantan Hospital, Capital Medical University, Beijing, P R China

References

[1] Barrow, D. L, Sector, R. H, Braun, I. F, Landmann, J. A, Tindall, S. C, & Tindall, G. T. (1985). Classification and treatment of spontaneous carotid cavernous fistula. J Neurosurg , 62, 248-256.

[2] Frechmann, N, Sartor, K, & Herrmann, H. D. (1981). Traumatic arteriovenous fistulae of the middle meningeal artery and neighbouring veins or dural sinuses. Acta Neurochir , 55, 273-281.

[3] Ishii, R, Ueki, K, & Ito, J. (1976). Traumatic fistula between a lacerated middle meningeal artery and a diploic vein: case report. J Neurosurg , 44, 241-244.

[4] Kawaguchi, T, Kawano, T, Kaneko, Y, Ooasa, T, Ooigawa, H, & Ogasawara, S. (2002). Traumatic lesions of the bilateral middle meningeal arteries-case report. Neurol Med Chir , 42, 221-223.

[5] Kitahara, T, Shirai, S, Owada, T, & Maki, Y. (1977). Traumatic middle meningeal arteriovenous fistula. Report of 3 cases and analysis of 32 cases. Eur Neurol , 16, 136-143.

[6] Matsumoto, K, Akagi, K, Abekura, M, & Tasaki, O. (2001). Vertex epidural hematoma associated with traumatic arteriovenous fistula of the middle meningeal artery: a case report. Surg Neurol , 55, 302-304.

[7] Roski, R. A, Owen, M, White, R. J, Takaoka, Y, & Ballon, E. M. (1982). Middle meningeal artery trauma. Surg Neurol , 17, 200-203.

[8] Sicat, L. C, Brinker, R. A, Abad, R. M, & Rovit, R. L. (1975). Traumatic pseudoaneurysm and arteriovenous fistula involving the middle meningeal artery. Surg Neurol , 3, 97-103.

[9] Bitoh, S, Hasegawa, H, Fujiwara, M, & Nakata, M. (1980). Traumatic arteriovenous fistula between the middle meningeal artery and cortical vein. Surg Neurol , 14, 355-358.

[10] Satoh, T, Sakurai, M, & Yamamoto, Y. Asaris((1983). Spontaneous closure of a traumatic middle meningeal arterio-venous fistula. Neuroradiology , 25, 105-109.

[11] Touho, H, Furuoka, N, Ohnishi, H, Komatsu, T, & Karasawa, J. (1995). Traumatic arteriovenous fistula treated by superselective embolization with microcoils:case report. Neuroradiology , 37, 65-67.

[12] Tsutsumi, M, Kazekawa, K, Tanaka, A, Ueno, Y, Nomoto, Y, Nii, K, & Harada, H. (2002). Traumatic middle meningeal artery pseudoaneurysm and subsequent fistula formation with the cavernous sinus. Surg Neurol , 58, 325-328.

[13] Debrun, G, Lacour, P, Caron, J. P, Hurth, M, Comoy, J, & Keravel, Y. (1978). Detachable balloon and calibrated-leak balloon techniques in the treatment of cerebral vascular lesions. J Neurosurg , 49, 635-49.

[14] Serbinenko, F. A. (1974). Balloon catheterization and occlusion of major cerebral vessels. J Neurosurg , 41, 125-45.

[15] Higashida, R. T, Halbach, V. V, Tsai, F. Y, Norman, D, Pribram, H. F, Mehringer, C. M, & Hieshima, G. B. (1989). Interventional neurovascular treatment of traumatic carotid and vertebral lesions: results in 234 cases. AJR AmJ Roentgenol , 153, 577-82.

[16] Debrun, G. M, Viñuela, F, Fox, A. J, Davis, K. R, & Ahn, H. S. (1988). Indications for treatment and classification of 132 carotid-cavernous fistulas. Neurosurgery , 22, 285-89.

[17] Lewis, A, & Tomsick, T. A. Tew JM Jr((1995). Management of 100 consecutive direct carotid-cavernous fistulas: results of treatment with detachable balloons. Neurosurgery , 36, 239-44.

[18] Tsai, Y. H, Wong, H. F, Chen, Y. L, & Weng, H. H. (2008). Transarterial Embolization of Direct Carotid Cavernous Fistulas with the Double-balloon Technique. Interv Neuroradiol. 14 Suppl , 2, 13-7.

[19] Naesens, R, Mestdagh, C, Breemersch, M, & Defreyne, L. (2006). Direct carotid-cavernous fistula: a case report and review of the literature. Bull Soc Belge Ophtalmol , 299, 43-54.

[20] Debrun, G, Lacour, P, Vinuela, F, Fox, A, Drake, C. G, & Caron, J. P. (1981). Treatment of 54 traumatic carotid-cavernous fistulas. J Neurosurg , 55, 678-92.

[21] Graeb, D. A, Robertson, W. D, Lapointe, J. S, & Nugent, R. A. (1985). Avoiding intra-arterial balloon detachment in the treatment of posttraumatic carotid-cavernous fistulae with detachable balloons. AJNR Am J Neuroradiol , 6, 602-05.

[22] Guglielmi, G, Viñuela, F, Briganti, F, & Duckwiler, G. (1992). Carotid-cavernous fistula caused by a ruptured intracavernous aneurysm: endovascular treatment by electrothrombosis with detachable coils. Neurosurgery , 31, 54-56.

[23] Siniluoto, T, Seppänen, S, Kuurne, T, Wikholm, G, Leinonen, S, & Svendsen, P. (1997). Transarterial embolization of a direct carotid cavernous fistula with Guglielmi detachable coils. AJNR Am J Neuroradiol , 18, 519-23.

[24] Seruga, T. (2006). Endovascular treatment of a direct post-traumatic carotid-cavernous fistula with electrolytically detachable coils. Wien Klin Wochenschr. 118 Suppl , 2, 80-4.

[25] Morón, F. E, Klucznik, R. P, Mawad, M. E, & Strother, C. M. (2005). Endovascular treatment of highflow carotid cavernous fistula by stent-assisted coil placement. AJNR Am J Neuroradiol , 26, 1399-404.

[26] Luo, C. B, Teng, M. M, Chang, F. C, & Chang, C. Y. (2006). Transarterial balloon-assisted n-butyl-2-cyanoacrylate embolization of direct carotid cavernous fistulas. AJNR Am J Neuroradiol , 27, 1535-40.

[27] Lv, X, Jiang, C, Li, Y, & Wu, Z. (2009). Percutaneous transvenous packing of cavernous sinus with Onyx for cavernous dural arteriovenous fistula. Eur J Radiol. , 71, 356-362.

[28] Zenteno, M, Santos-franco, J, Rodríguez-parra, V, Balderrama, J, Aburto-murrieta, Y, Vega-montesinos, S, & Lee, A. (2010). Management of direct carotid-cavernous sinus fistulas with the use of ethylene-vinyl alcohol [Onyx] only: preliminary results. J Neurosurg. , 112, 595-602.

[29] Tsai, Y. H, Wong, H. F, Weng, H. H, & Chen, Y. L. (2010). Comparison of the risk of oculomotor nerve deficits between detachable balloons and coils in the treatment of direct carotid cavernous fistulas. AJNR Am J Neuroradiol. , 31, 1123-6.

[30] Gökalp, H. Z, & Ozkal, E. (1979). Surgical treatment of traumatic carotid cavernous fistulas. Clin Neurol Neurosurg. 1979;, 81, 130-4.

[31] Lin, C. J, Luo, C. B, Chang, F. C, Teng, M. M, Wang, K. L, & Chu, S. H. (2009). Combined transarterial, transvenous, and direct puncture of the cavernous sinus to cure a traumatic carotid cavernous fistula. J Clin Neurosci. , 16, 1663-5.

[32] Jiang, C, Lv, X, Li, Y, Wu, Z, & Shi, J. Surgical access on the superior ophthalmic vein to the cavernous sinus dural fistula for embolization. J Neurointerv Surg. doi: 10.1136/neurintsurg-

Section 5

Iatrogenic Arteriovenous Fistula

Chapter 12

Arterialized Venous Flaps in Reconstructive and Plastic Surgery

Hede Yan, Cunyi Fan, Feng Zhang and Weiyang Gao

Additional information is available at the end of the chapter

http://dx.doi.org/10.5772/56364

1. Introduction

Venous flaps are defined as a composite flap of skin and subcutaneous veins that relies on the venous system alone for flap perfusion, that is, the primary blood supply enters and exits the flap through the venous system. [1] Unlike conventional arterial flaps, venous flaps do not sacrifice an artery of the donor site nor do they require deep dissection. This results in an easier procedure as well as a decrease in morbidity of the donor site. In addition, they are thinner and more pliable because they consist only of skin, venous plexus, and subcutaneous fat. They can also be transferred simultaneously as a composite flap to reconstruct the defects of affected tendons and vessels. [2]- [9] These advantages make venous flaps an ideal indication for the repair of soft tissue defects in hands and fingers, especially when the local flaps and other conventional flaps are not available. [10]

The arterialized venous flaps (AVFs) were first introduced in an experimental study by Nakayama et al in 1981 [1] and in clinical practice in 1987. [11], [12] Since then, during the last decades the AVFs have been mainly utilized in reconstructive surgeries as a result of more unreliable outcomes of early clinical studies using purely venous flaps with venous inflow and outflow. [13] In the early clinical study, Yoshimura et al transplanted 13 flaps with arterial inflow and venous outflow. Twelve flaps survived completely; one had superficial necrosis leading the authors to confirm that arterialized venous flaps were more reliable.

However, many problems have also been encountered using this flap in clinical settings, especially in several relatively large series. [9], [14]- [16] Lorenzi et al [15] noted that postoperative congestion was present in all flaps; partial necrosis rate was as high as 42.5 % with a total flap necrosis rate of 7.5 %; a superficial epidermolysis occurred in 17.5% of flaps causing the development of a full-thickness skin necrosis that required grafting. Inoue et al [14] demonstrated that failure rates as high as 50% occurred in 15 patients when a large arterialized venous flap from the leg was used. A subsequent series involving 16 arterialized venous flaps showed some improvement of flap survival, but the outcomes were still not satisfactory with only seven complete successes, six partial successes, and three complete failures.

Due to the unpredictable survivals of the arterialized venous flaps, many modifications have been practiced in an attempt to improve its survival status, including flap design, venous orientation, venous anatomy, and using noncontiguous central veins. [17] Undoubtedly, certain improvements on the application of all kinds of AVFs have been achieved; however, many questions are still left unanswered.

2. Animal models for experimental investigations of AVFs

Since high occurrence rate of partial flap necrosis and prolonged healing or secondary procedures, further investigation is needed for this non-conventional flap. Several animal models have been developed for experimental studies with the involvement of rats, rabbits, dogs and pigs as well.

The first animal model developed for the study of venous flaps was the rat reported by Nakayama et al in 1981. [1] The flap was designed using the superficial inferior epigastric vein distally and a branch of the lateral thoracic vein proximally served as the venous system. The arterialized venous flap model was established with the anastomosis between the epigastic vein in the flap and the femoral artery in the distal side. Lenoble and associates [18] described another venous flap, which was sited transversely between the left and right epigastric venous systems.

Rabbits are the most common animal model utilized for the study of venous flaps. [18]- [24] The rabbit ear has served as a model for venous flaps. Its reliable anatomic characteristics have provided additional rationale for the selection of this model making this flap a genuine flow-through venous flap. Another model for the venous flap in rabbits was illustrated by Xiu et al. [25] The venous flap was tailored along the axis of the thoracoepigastic veins as a flow-through venous flap. Recently, Tan et al [24] introduced another rabbit model for the evaluation of retrograde flow venous flaps. Although clinical and experimental studies have concentrated mainly on the antegrade arterialization of venous flaps to increase survival, retrograde AVFs may have the greatest potential. This animal model utilized the rabbit's valved, thoracoepigastric vein (consisting of the lateral thoracic and epigastric veins) as the source vessel for the study of retrograde arterialized venous flaps (RAVFs). This designed rabbit thoracoepigastric RAVF is simple to apply and easily reproducible. It is the first animal flap adapted specifically for the study of RAVFs, and may be used for the further investigation of these flaps, which have shown unpredictable survival to date.

There are also several other animal models undertaken as venous flap models, which were not widely utilized in experimental studies, including the dog saphenous or cephalic venous flaps [26] and the swine pedicled buttock venous flap [27].

3. Mechanisms of flap survival

Arterialized venous flaps differ from conventional flaps in that the classic Harvesian model of arterial inflow-capillaries-venous outflow is replaced by the arterial inflow- without capillary network-venous outflow. There are considerable controversies on the real nature of their survivals accompanied with their advent. Investigations on the blood supply of venous flaps mostly focus on the purely venous flaps. [26], [28], [29]

Noreldin et al [28] performed an experimental study to investigate how the perivenous areolar tissue affects survival of the rat inferior epigastric venous flap model in 1992. Histological examination of the pedicle showed that many minute vascular channels (single-cell-layered capillaries) were present apart from the inferior epigastric vein. This result confirms the importance of the perivenous areolar tissue in perfusion of the skin island, at least, in the inferior epigastric venous flap in the rat. In another study from Shalaby et al [29], histological study of the pedicles of long and short saphenous and cephalic venous flaps in fresh human cadavers and two clinical cases showed that one or two arterioles and multiple capillaries were present in the perivenous areolar tissue, indicating the perivenous areolar tissue which contains small arteries is vital to the survival of venous flaps in rats.

On the other hand, the results of Xiu et al's showed that the similar perivenous areolar tissue was purely venous and had no fine arteries with the vein in the rabbit, and the role of perivenous areolar tissue is strictly to protect and nourish the vein itself. They otherwise proved that the profuse venous network in flow-through venous flaps and early invasion of new blood vessels are the mainstays of venous flap survival. [25] Another hypothesis of "to-and-fro" flow [26] was also introduced as the single venous channels providing both perfusion and drainage to the flap tissue, and the "to-and-fro" flow in the single vein was also observed. Many authors demonstrated that the early invasion of new blood vessels is essential to venous flap survival and the low perfusion of venous flaps enhances the invasion of new vessels. [25]

Whatever hypotheses of its survival mechanisms were put forward, three main theories have been postulated as to the physiology of the venous flap. These include "A-V shunting" or retrograde flow from the venous system to the arterial system via paralyzed arterial-venous shunts, "reverse flow" or flow from the venules into the capillaries, and "capillary bypass" or flow through the venous system without entrance into the arterial side until neovascularization. [30] There is no conclusive evidence and therefore no consensus regarding the exact mechanism for venous flap survival. However, it is probable that a combined work of the aforementioned factors is responsible for the perfusion of venous flaps and further investigation is required for better understanding of its survival mechanisms.

4. Classifications

In literature, several classification systems have been developed and still being updated. It is essential to gain insight into its classifications based on the fully understanding of this flap, facilitating promising clinical outcomes.

The classification of venous flaps utilized in clinical setting was first introduced by Chen and colleagues in 1991. [31] In their original report, venous flaps were classified into four types: Type I, a free venous flap with total venous perfusion where both ends of its vein was anastomosed with two veins; Type II, a pedicled venous flap with total venous perfusion where one end of the vein was intact and the other end of the vein was anastomosed to an adjacent vein; Type III, a free venous flap of arterialized venous perfusion with an afferent A-V fistula where the distal anastomosis was an artery to a vein and the proximal anastomosis was a vein to a vein; Type IV, a venous flap with total arterialized venous perfusion in which both ends of the vein were connected to arteries. Type I and II flaps have a failure rate between 30 and 80% and are limited to small flaps. [17] It is postulated that their poor survival is due to the low O_2 concentration of the afferent blood supply and venous congestion. [30] Type III and type IV are the basic patterns of arterialized venous flaps. The author didn't emphasize the concerns of intravenous valve in their classification system; however, it is supposed that both types of arterialized venous flaps are perfused in an antegrade mode based on their illustrations. Although Arterialized venous flaps show higher survival rates than type I or II venous flaps, they are still prone to venous congestion and partial full-thickness necrosis. [10], [32] (Figure 1)

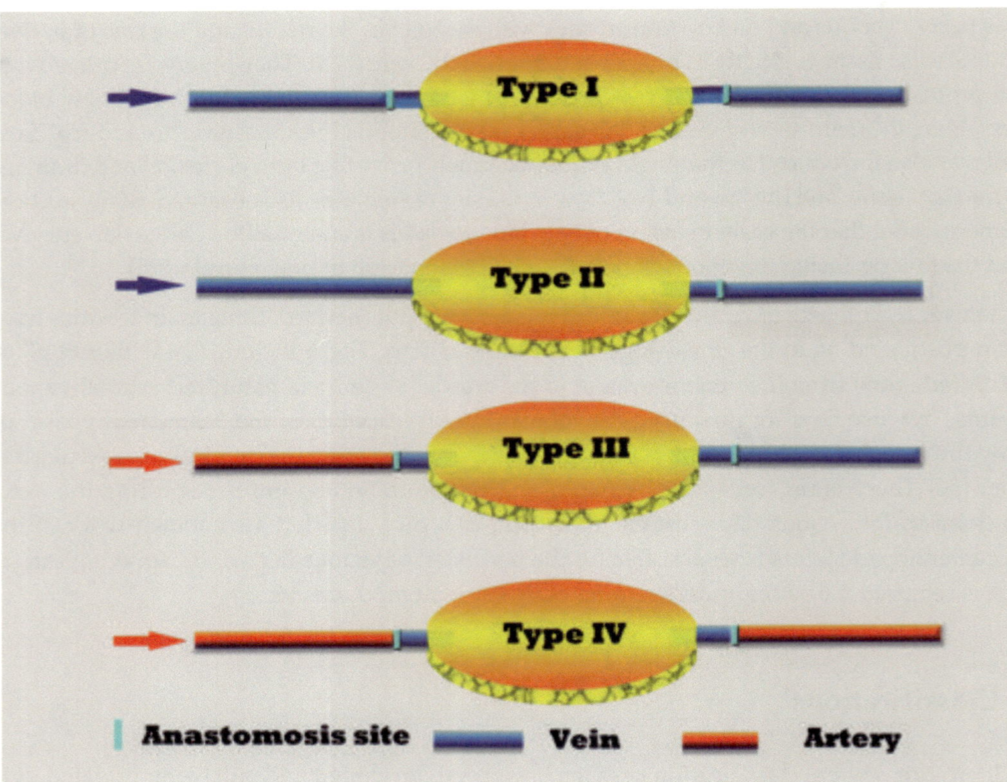

Figure 1.

Thereafter, Thatte et al [33] proposed a three-type classification system of venous flaps. This classification, which was based on the vessels that enter and leave the flap as well as the direction of flow within these vessels, was detailed as follows: type I, unipedicled venous flaps; type II, bipedicled venous flaps; type III, arterio-venous venous flaps. This classification system briefly illustrates the general modes of venous flaps which were cited most commonly both experimentally and clinically. Then In 1994, Fukui et al [34] proposed another four-type classification system of venous flaps, which is very similar to that of Chen et al's. In 2007, Woo et al [35] refined the classification of arterialized venous flaps used in hand and finger reconstruction into three types. Their classification takes into consideration the presence of an intravenous valve, the venous network of the donor site, the location, and the number of veins at the recipient site. Type I is a "through and along-valve" type which mimics similar blood flow as in a standard vein graft with a straight or Y-shaped pattern. Type II is against-valve, which is arterial inflow against the valve through the afferent vein with a reversed Y- or H-shaped venous network. In type III venous flaps, venous flow drains through efferent veins against intravenous valves. (Figure 2)

Recently, Goldschlager et al [17] further modified the flow-through venous flaps, which were also divided into four types: type I and type II are the same to Chen's classification; type III) and IV) are arterialized flaps, similar as described by Chen et al. However, two descriptors were added: C_x, the number of efferent vessels contiguous with the central vein, where "x" refers to the number of central efferent vessels with zero included; and P_x, the number of efferent veins discontiguous with the central vein, where "x" refers to the number of peripheral efferent vessels with zero included. The direction of flow is assumed to be along the valve, unless the descriptor "retrograde" is added. In this classification system as shown above, the following concerns were considered: 1) the type of afferent vessel anastomosed to the central vein, 2) the type of efferent vessel anastomosed to the central vein, 3) the number of efferent vessels, 4) the number of efferent veins that are not contiguous with the central vein, that is the number of peripheral veins, 5) whether the central vein is pedicled or not, either at the afferent or at the efferent end, and 6) the direction of the central vein. So far, this classification system provides a simple and descriptive nomenclature for venous flaps. (Figure 3)

5. Clinical applications

5.1. Resurfacing of skin defects only in hand surgery

Arterialized venous flaps have been mostly used for the closure of small defects, especially on hand and digits. Yoshimura et al. [11] first introduced the arterialized venous flap in 1987. Thirteen arterialized venous flaps measuring in size from 1.3 cm x 3.1 cm to 6.0 cm x 1.0 cm were utilized to resurface the skin defects at fingers in 11 cases. Complete survival was achieved in 12 (92.3%) and 1 sustained partial superficial necrosis. Later, they presented another larger series of these flaps for the coverage of skin defects on the hands in 22 patients, of which an A-V-A type of venous flap was used in 12 patients and an A-V-V type in 10 patients. [36] Seventeen were completely successful, 4 were partially

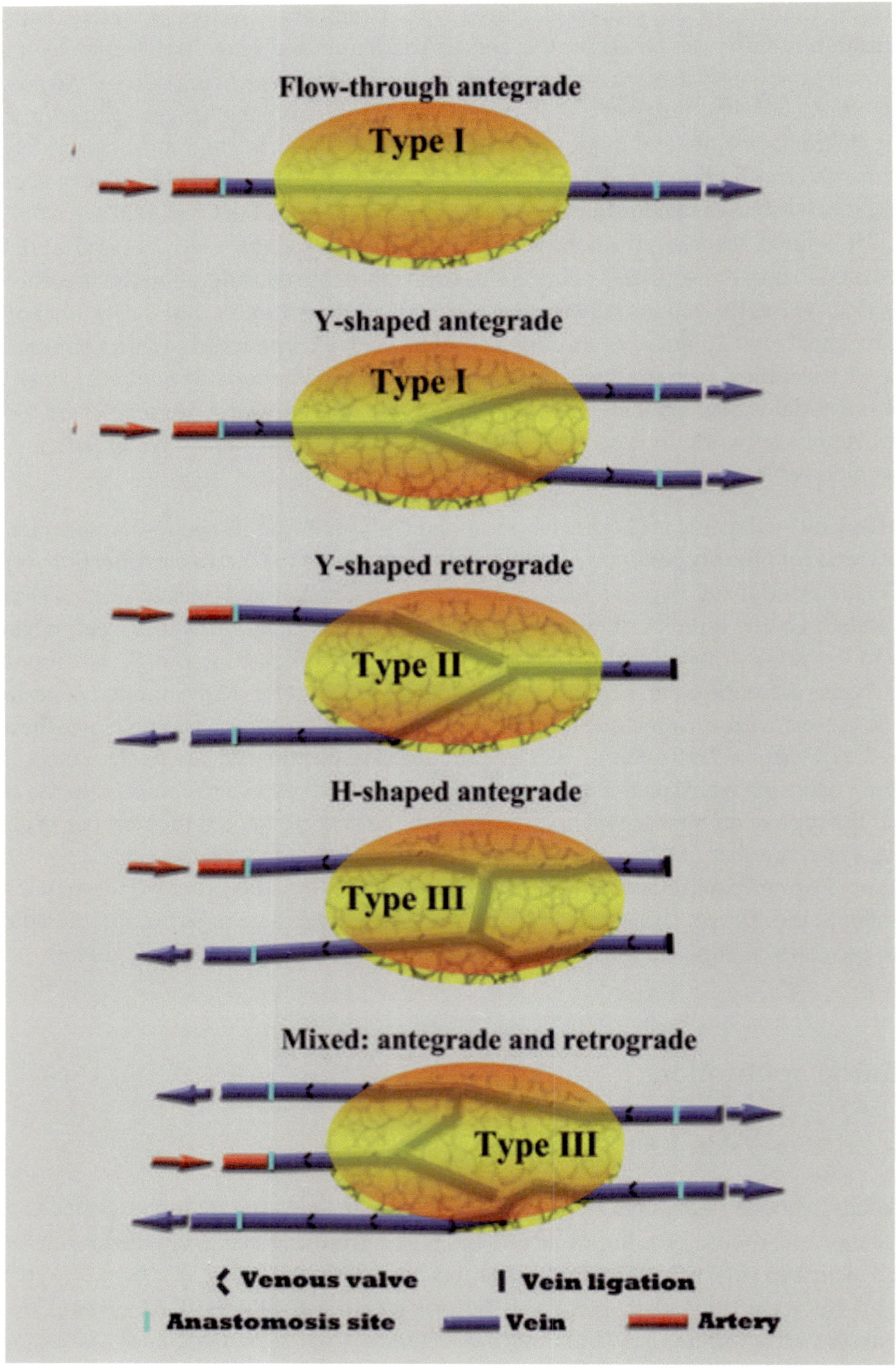
Flow-through antegrade
Type I
Y-shaped antegrade
Type I
Y-shaped retrograde
Type II
H-shaped antegrade
Type III
Mixed: antegrade and retrograde
Type III
Venous valve
Vein ligation
Anastomosis site
Vein
Artery

Figure 2.

http://dx.doi.org/10.5772/56364

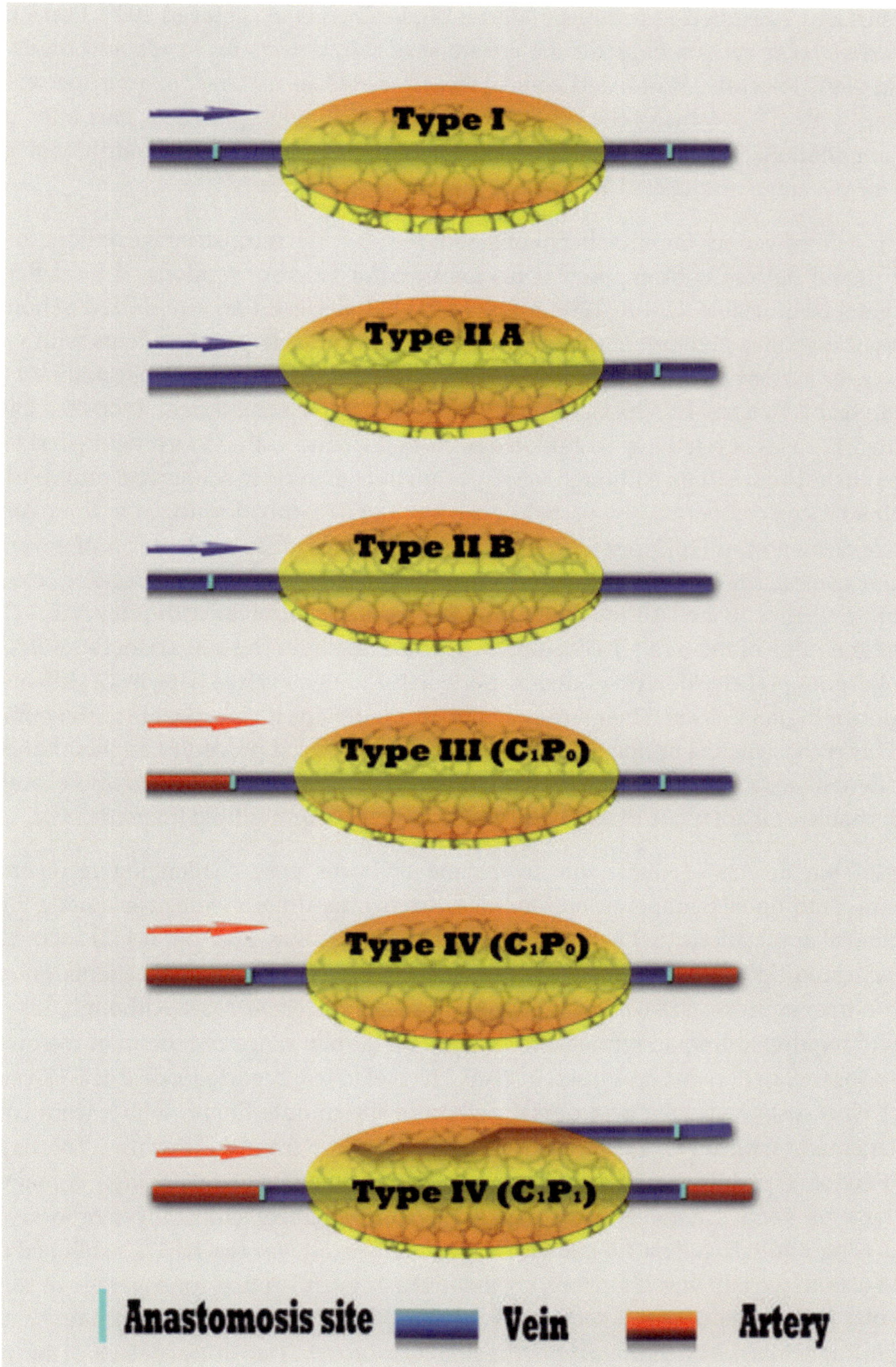

Figure 3.

successful and 1 resulted in complete failure. While Chen et al achieved 100% flap survival using arterialized venous flaps for the coverage of skin defects on hands and digits in 11 cases in 1991. Recently, Brook and colleagues succeeded in resurfacing an upper extremity stump with a 9 x 6-cm venous flap harvested from a nonreplantable part after partial hand amputation. The flap provided durable coverage, and avoided additional procedures for coverage and staged tendon reconstructions. [37]

The Arterialized venous flaps has been considered as potential reconstructive options for large dorsal digital defects with exposed bone, joint and/or extensor tendons, if local flaps are inadequate or unusable. [10] In 1996, Yilmaz et al [38] designed an arterialized venous flap utilizing the venous network of the forearm and applied this flap in 5 patients with various defects in the extremities ranging in size from 6 x 8 cm to 10 x 12 cm. Four flaps totally survived. One flap had 30% partial necrosis. Overall clinical results were successful. Woo et al [39] also presented 12 cases of relatively large skin defects of the hand with AVFs ranging in size from 6 cm x 3 cm to 14 cm x 9 cm. Although the flaps showed remarkable edema and multiple bullae on their surface postoperatively, partial necrosis of the flap only developed in three cases. In 2004, Nakazawa et al [40] presented four cases of successful reconstruction of severe and extensive contractures of the palm using large arterialized venous flaps measuring from 5 cm x 13 cm to 9 cm x 17 cm. All four flaps showed complete survival with uneventful clinical courses and none of them required a defatting procedure after the operation. Recently, Hyza and colleagues [41] also described their experience of 13 venous free flaps in 12 patients with large dorsal digital defects. Their survival rate for these flaps is comparable to the published data. This reconstructive option has become a well-established procedure in their hands and is the alternate reconstructive method of choice for large dorsal digital defects where local flaps are not usable or inadequate due to complex hand injuries or multiple finger defects.

Multiple skin defects of digits due to trauma or burns pose challenging reconstructive problems. Traditional therapeutic options for salvaging these digits were problematic, limiting their clinical applications to the treatment of injury. Inoue G and Suzuki K [42] succeeded in resurfacing multiple skin defects of hand caused by trauma or burns in five patients. Four flaps survived uneventfully (80%), and 1 showed 30 percent partial necrosis. Although this procedure will require additional refinement, it permits a certain range of motion of the involved digits prior to flap division and inset. In 2005, Hyza et al [43] reported a case of a 17-year-old patient who sustained volar and dorsal defects of the middle finger, which were covered simultaneously with bilobed arterialized venous free flap from the forearm. The flap was composed of 2 paddles, which were connected by a subcutaneous bridge containing a subcutaneous venous network. The flap survived completely with only temporary mild venous congestion. Excellent functional and cosmetic result was reached. The bilobed arterialized venous free flap was, therefore, considered as a useful option for coverage of concomitant volar and dorsal digital defects. Trovato et al [44] also treated a patient who sustained multiple finger injuries on the hand with the similar approach. Two dorsal defects of the middle and ring fingers were covered simultaneously with a single arterialized venous free flap from the right forearm. The flap was used to create a dorsally syndactylized digit which survived completely and was subsequently divided longitudinally. The key point for the coverage of

http://dx.doi.org/10.5772/56364

multiple defects in fingers with this flap is to select the proper donor site, in which a sufficient diffuse venous plexus and lax configuration including at least two separate pathways for anastomosing with the recipient vessels should be ensured. [10] Therefore, this application of Arterialized venous flaps is a useful option for the simultaneous coverage of multiple skin defects of digits and excellent functional and cosmetic results can be expected.

5.2. Reconstruction of both skin and vascular defects in hand surgery

Due to the anatomical nature of venous flaps, the best scenario for the clinical use of the arterialized venous flap occurs when both revascularisation and skin coverage are needed. [10] Honda et al [13] first developed the clinical application of the arterialized venous flap as a composite skin and subcutaneous vein graft in the replantation of six amputated digits which were complicated by the loss of skin and veins and with the exposure of bone and tendon in 1984. Satisfactory results were obtained. Then in 1989, Nishi et al [2] reported seven cases of arterialized venous flaps for the treatment of both skin and digital arterial defects. The flaps were applied to cover the skin defect as well as to restore blood circulation. Almost complete survival of the flaps was achieved in all cases. In 1993, Fasika et al [3] also achieved the similar outcomes in their series. In 1999, Koch et al [5] reported the first case of successful coverage of a skin and soft-tissue defect, including revascularization with an arterialized venous flap bridging both arterial and venous defects in a finger avulsion injury. Similarly, several other case reports with this flap for the same purpose all achieved satisfactory results, [4], [45], [46] indicating that this procedure is a well-established technique to not only provide flap coverage for exposed bone and tendon, but also provide an one-stage procedure for digits in need of revascularization and skin coverage.

5.3. Reconstruction of both skin and tendon defects in hand surgery

It is not rare that composite components defects including extensor tendons can occur simultaneously in clinical settings and the treatment will become extremely challenging, especially when multiple fingers are involved. Ideally, surgical management of these defects should fulfill the goal of primary reconstruction in a single surgical procedure with thin and reliable flaps. Conventionally, these injuries are managed with primary soft tissue coverage followed by a later secondary tendon reconstruction. In literature, local or regional flaps are often the preferred choice for soft tissue reconstruction of hand and digits; however, when facing larger dorsal defects, extensive and multiple digits injuries, these flaps are sometimes precluded and free flaps are frequently considered as the optimal options. In 1991, Inoue and Tamura [6] first introduced a novel technique of composite free-flap and tendon transfer using an arterialized venous flap containing the palmaris longus tendon to repair finger injuries involving the skin and both flexor and extensor tendons in four patients. Although the final range of motion was disappointing, with an average of 10 degrees, further trials of this technique conducted in four more patients achieved encouraging results after refining the indications of the procedure. [47] In 1994, Chen et al [7] reported three similar cases of combined skin and tendon loss on the dorsum of the finger that were treated with the same procedure and achieved good results. Their investigations demonstrated that the technique is feasible and offers a good treatment modality for the small but complex defects on the dorsum of the finger using a one-stage operation. [10]

Then In 1999, Cho et al [8] introduced a similar technique which was applied to reconstruct the defects of skin and multiple extensor tendons on the dorsum of hand using Arterialized venous flaps in a manner of surgical delay in two cases. The patients were reconstructed with a dorsalis pedis tendocutaneous arterialized venous flap. One patient sustained a soft-tissue defect on the dorsum of the right hand, including the absence of the extensor pollicis longus and the extensor digitorum communis of the index finger, and the other sustained a soft-tissue defect on the dorsum of the right hand with the absence of the extensor digitorum communis tendons of the index and middle fingers. Two weeks after the surgical delay on the donor site, an arterialized venous flap, including the extensor digitorum longus tendons of the second and third toes, was transferred to the recipient site. Excellent results were achieved both aesthetically and functionally. Although this technique is a two-stage operation with donor-site scarring and weak extension of the toes, a larger arterialized venous flap can be obtained than when using a pure venous flap or arterialized venous flap; this technique also can increase the survival rate, and multiple tendon grafts can be harvested simultaneously. [10]

Recently, we performed 7 composite palmaris longus venous flaps and 5 arterialized venous flaps with an average size of 6.1cm x 2.9 cm in the reconstruction of post-traumatic extensive dorsal digital injuries in 8 patients. [48] All the flaps survived completely despite of the occurrence of universal venous congestion and swelling. The outcomes at an average follow-up of about 12 months were very satisfactory in terms of functional recovery, aesthetic appearance and sensation restoration. Based on our experience, the Arterialized venous flaps are reliable and good candidates for resurfacing large dorsal digital defects when local flaps are not available or insufficient for coverage. Composite arterialized venous flap with palmaris longus tendon is an optimal choice for one-stage reconstruction of dorsal composite finger injuries.

5.4. Innervated arterialized venous flap

Sensation is vital to hand function and it is always optimal to resurface a skin defect and reconstruct the sensation simultaneously whenever possible. In 1998, Kayikcioglu et al [49] first reported two cases using innervated Arterialized venous flaps and achieved satisfactory sensory recovery with 4 - 6 mm static two-point discrimination. They concluded that the innervated arterialized venous flap is a useful method that provides functional and cosmetic coverage for digit reconstruction. Then in 2000, Takeuchi et al [50] presented two more innervated arterialized venous flaps for the reconstruction of finger degloving injuries from the dorsum of the foot. Sensation was preserved by anastomosing branches of superficial peroneal nerves with the digital nerves. All the flaps provided successful coverage over the denuded fingers. Good sensation and nearly full range of motion of the fingers were obtained. In our study we also found that all the innervated AVFs for the fingertip reconstruction almost obtained normal sensation at a mean follow-up of 15.4 months, while most cases of the insensate AVFs only achieved protective sensation. Cold intolerance was present in most cases of the insensate group in comparison with the sensate group with only one case suffering from slight cold intolerance. [51] However, Kushima et al [52] revealed that the sensory recovery was satisfactory even without nerve repair in the application of this flap. Their study hypothesized that the sensory recovery after AVFs transfer on hand and digits was donor-site dependent without nerve repair. In their serial, soft tissue loss of fingers were repaired in 22 patients using 25 arterialized venous flaps harvested from the thenar, hypothenar, or forearm regions. Good sensory recovery was obtained for the thenar and hypothenar venous flaps, while moving two-point discrimination was not recorded during the follow-up period in the group using forearm venous flaps. Therefore, the differences among these studies regarding the sensation recovery after reconstruction with AVFs in hand surgery can't be single factor of nerve repairing dependent and most possibly they are as a work of multiple factors, like donor sites, recipient sites, patients' demographic disparities, etc.

5.5. Reconstruction of degloving injuries in hand surgery

Circumferential defects of the digits are uncommon but present a challenging problem to the surgeons. Although many reconstructive options are available for the treatment of this injury, simple skin grafting tends to cause tendon adhesions, limiting the range of motion. The use of local skin flaps, such as a cross-finger flap, is limited by the considerable skin loss that is naturally found in a defect that is circumferential in nature. Other options include the use of a reversed forearm flap or some free tissue transfers resulting in limited donor sites available as well as donor morbidity. [53] Takeuchi et al [50] first described the technique of the reconstruction of digit avulsion injuries with arterialized venous flaps in a wrap-around fashion in 2000. Chia et al reported another case in which the circumferential defect of an index finger, measuring 6 cm around the digit and 3 cm long, is resurfaced by the use of a free arterialized venous flap raised from the volar forearm skin with excellent contour and full range of motion. Recently, Brook et al [54] presented use of the this flap for the reconstruction of severe ring avulsion injury. Eight AVFs were transplanted for 3 Urbaniak class II and 5 Urbaniak class III ring avulsions. Average size of the venous flap was 6 cm^2. All flaps and digits survived without partial necrosis. The soft tissue envelope was supple in all cases. Total active motion (TAM) ranged from 160 to 210 degrees. Based on all these results, the arterialized venous flap has proven itself to be a reliable solution for the complex circumferential avulsion injury which requires simultaneous soft tissue and digital vessel reconstruction. [10]

5.6. Reconstruction of finger pulp

Fingertip injuries also pose a challenging reconstructive problem. Various skin flaps have been used in the reconstruction of fingertip defects. In repairing pulp tissue loss, local flaps are the first choice from the point of view of sensory recovery and skin texture. In cases where local flaps are not suitable, regional flaps harvested from elsewhere in the hand, such as the cross-finger flap or the thenar flap, are applied. However, these methods require long immobilization, multiple operations, and lengthy hospitalizations. [10] Iwasawa et al [55] introduced a new fingertip reconstruction procedure with arterialized venous flaps from the thenar or hypothenar regions. In their study, 13 of the 15 flaps survived completely. All the flaps that survived exhibited stable coverage and good texture at follow-up. These flaps are not sensory flaps; however, they exhibited useful sensory recovery within 6 months of the operation. This showed that the thenar and hypothenar skin is durable with appropriate texture for replacement of fingertip defects. However, this donor site is size limited and the conspicuous scaring might be a concern at follow up, especially when primary closure can be achieved. Yokoyama et al [56]- [58] developed the medial plantar area as a donor site for AVFs in the reconstruction of large finger pulp defect. The medial plantar venous flap was designed, the distal subcutaneous vein or communicating vein of the medial plantar area was anastomosed to the proper digital artery, and the proximal vein of the flap was anastomosed to the dorsal subcutaneous vein of the stump of the digit. The flaps survived in all the patients. At 12 months after the surgery, all the treated fingers had attained a good shape and sensory restoration. We also found that the survival of AVFs harvested from the medial plantar area was more "natural" than from the forearm without obvious edema and venous congestion. (Figure 4 a-h vs Figure 5 a-h)

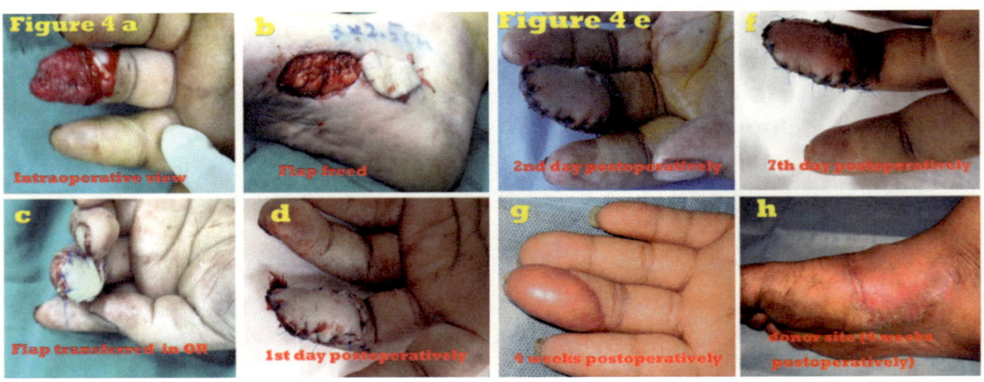

Figure 4.

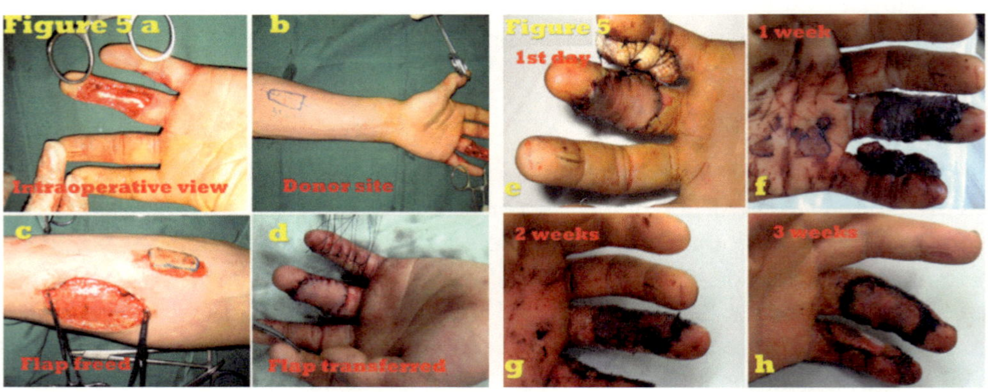

Figure 5.

http://dx.doi.org/10.5772/56364

5.7. Reconstruction of fingernails

The reconstruction of a missing or deficient nail is an important and difficult procedure for plastic surgeons. The vascularized free graft is becoming increasingly reliable, and it is now considered to be the best method. [59] However, preparation of the vascularized nail graft is rather difficult and tedious. To simplify this procedure, Nakayama et al [60] developed a new method to reconstruct the fingernails using the principles from the arterialized venous flaps in 1990. Three patients underwent successful transplantation of the great toenails to their index fingers utilizing the venous system of the nail graft for perfusion by anatomosing the two venous pedicles with the recipient digital artery and dorsal vein. Then in 1999, Patradul et al reported ten arterialized venous toenail flaps for the reconstruction of fingernail loss due to trauma in nine patients. Four flaps were taken from the lateral part of the big toe and six flaps from the second toe. Four toenail flaps with pulp and three flaps with the distal half of distal phalanx were used. Nine flaps survived completely and one had partial necrosis. All showed excellent aesthetic and functional results except for one case with minimal deformity in growth of the nail. They suggested that this procedure is easy, reliable, and a useful alternative for the reconstruction of nail loss.

5.8. Resurfacing soft tissue defects other than hand and digits

Based on the special nature of venous flaps, their applications have not been limited for the reconstruction of soft tissue defects in hand and digits only. In 1998, Kovacs [61] first utilized this kind of flaps for oral reconstruction with varied results. In 2008, Iglesias et al [62] used a forearm arterialized venous free flap (23 cm x 14 cm) in a 25-year-old male with facial burns sequels to reconstruct both cheeks, chin, lips, nose, columnella, nasal tip, and nostrils. It was arterialized by the facial artery to an afferent vein anastomosis. The venous flow was drained by four efferent vein to vein anastomoses. Although it developed small inferior marginal necrosis in the lower lip, the rest of the flap survived with good quality of the skin in both texture and color without the need of additional thinning surgical procedures.

After extensive excision of skin cancer on the face, or when skin cancer is located on the 3-dimensional structures of the face, reconstruction with a local flap can be impossible, or clinicians are reluctant to reconstruct defects with a skin graft because of postoperative contraction, hyperpigmentation, or other complication. Instead, an arterialized venous free flap can be used as an alternative method of reconstruction to prevent distortion and recurrence. [63]

Recently, Park and colleagues [63] reported eight patients underwent surgery with an arterialized venous-free flap. All of the soft-tissue defects made by excising the tumor were reconstructed with good outcomes, except for 1 case. Regarding the cosmetic evaluation, the color was fair, the contour and texture were good, absence of distortion of surrounding structures was excellent, and the overall results in most all cases were good. There were no recurrences or metastases during the follow-up period. They considered that the arterialized venous flap is an alternative plan among several reconstruction methods when skin cancer on the face is extensively excised.

6. Surgical principles

The arterialized venous flap is an unconventional flap in that the classic Harvesian model of arterial inflow-capillaries-venous outflow is replaced by the venous inflow-capillary network-venous outflow. The physiological basis for its survival is not entirely understood. Due to its atypical pattern as a skin flap, its progress is not easily predictable. Generally, the following concepts are regarded as guidelines for the design of arterialized venous flaps: (1) avoid perfusing the afferent phase by applying the largest possible arterial flow; (2) lax configuration of the efferent phase, using at least two available receptor veins; and (3) flap designing over the diffuse venous plexus while attempting to include not only the pathway of a single vein. Furthermore, the following principles are of great importance for success: firstly, the afferent vein must be left close to the recipient artery in order to avoid pedicle kinking; and secondly, the efferent veins must be longer in order to reach the recipient veins. [64]

Inoue et al [14] observed that the survival status of AVFs appeared to be influenced by the donor site and size of the flap. When a small flap from the forearm was used, the success rate was almost 100 percent. However, there was a 50 percent success rate when a large flap from the leg was used. Recently, Kakinoki et al [65] performed a retrospective analysis of the free arterialized venous flaps that were utilized in 51 patients to identify prognostic factors that correlate with flap necrosis. Multivariate analysis showed that the size of the flap was the factor that correlated statistically with a successful result after a flap operation. They found that the arterialized venous flaps that were less likely to develop necrosis of the skin generally had a surface area less than 767 mm^2. The influence of donor site on the survival of arterialized venous flaps may be attributed to the configuration of venous network of different donor sites. This postulation has also been revealed in our practice. (Figure 4 a-h vs Figure 5 a-h) Of all the popular donor sites for arterialized venous flaps, it is believed that the configuration of the dorsal skin of digits and hypothenar or thenar is more favorable than that of the volar forearm, while the donor site of lower leg, in which there is a poor venous network, is considered the last choice for venous flaps. On the other hand, the medial plantar area might be the optimal donor site for the reconstruction of the finger pulp defect in terms of functional and cosmetic concerns together with the consideration of donor site morbidities.

7. Technical controversies

7.1. Type III vs Type IV

Basically two perfusion patterns are related to the AVFs, that is, either Chen's [31] or Goldschlager's [17] type III (A-V-V) and type IV (A-V-A). The investigation of Nishi et al's [16] showed that type IV is likely more favorable than type III. Based on most of the literature that was reviewed, however, no significant difference in flap survival rate was noted despite that the statistical analysis was precluded. [10] The A-V-A type is mostly used for skin coverage and providing a conduit for arterial flow when the vessel is injured. The A-V-V type can be used regardless of the location of the soft tissue defect and therefore has been more widely used. The A-V-V type has been used in many situations including multiple digits, fingertip, finger shaft injuries, web space, and circumferential soft tissue defects.

7.2. Antegrade vs retrograde

A majority of AVFs used in clinical practice were applied in an antegrade perfusion fashion. However, controversies were put forward in an attempt to demonstrate that retrograde perfusion can enhance the perfusion of the flaps. [10] An experimental study with flaps from human cadavers indicated that blood circulation in the periphery of arterialized venous flaps can be increased by retrograde arterialization. [66] Koch et al [67] utilized the retrograde arterialized venous flaps to resurface the skin and soft-tissue defects in 13 flaps. There was venous congestion with superficial epidermolysis in six flaps, but not in the other seven. All flaps survived except for partial skin necrosis in two of the lower-extremity flaps. Their results suggest that retrograde perfusion enhances blood flow in the periphery of arterialized venous flaps and gives good results in terms of flap survival, especially on the upper extremity. They speculated that if blood flows through the flap in the original anatomic direction, and thus the venous valves do not impose any resistance to blood flow. As a result, the greater part of the blood flows through the flap's central vein only and that the flap's periphery will be in danger of insufficient perfusion leading to partial necrosis. While Woo et al [35] recently also published their clinical series utilizing their antegrade approach with a 98% (151/154) success rate and a 5.2% (8/154) partial loss rate. These studies show that either antegrade or retrograde approach can result in success rates comparable to conventional flaps. However, few further investigations were found in literature using the retrograde arterialized venous flaps in clinical setting, so caution should be taken for clinical applications. [10]

8. Technical modifications

8.1. Delay procedures

Surgical delay procedures have been researched and applied clinically in traditional flap transfers to extend the expected survival length of a flap, to define the survival of a flap of uncertain viability, and to improve the circulation of an established flap of expected viability. [68] Byun et al [22] first reported that a14-day delay procedure significantly increased the survival of arterialized venous flaps with a 94.0 % of mean viable surface area of the flaps in the delayed group compared to total necrosis in the non-delayed group. Subsequently, Cho et al [20] investigated the efficacy of a surgical delay procedure and a combined surgical and chemical delay procedure on the survival of arterialized venous flaps. The mean percentage survival of arterialized venous flaps was from 36.6 % to 59.7 % in different period delay groups, while in the combined surgical and chemical delay group, the mean percentage survival was on average 90 %. They concluded that the combination of surgical and chemical delay procedures would be more effective than any of the single delay procedures in increasing the survival of arterialized venous flaps, and the delay period could be shortened.

In clinical practice, arterialized venous flaps using delay procedures were first reported by Cho et al [69] in 1997 and achieved satisfactory results. They reported a series of 15 flaps using surgical or surgical-chemical delay procedure with only one flap loss. Their results suggest that except for a disadvantage of two-stage operation, the delayed arterialized venous flap may develop a larger flap than can be obtained with a pure venous flap or arterialized venous flap and increase the survival rate of the arterialized venous flap, which permits the possibility of using a composite flap besides all the advantages of the pure venous flap.

8.2. Pre-arterialization techniques

Pre-arterialization is considered as a promising procedure to improve the survival of venous flaps and this concept was first introduced by Nakayama et al [1]. Briefly, pre-arterialization was achieved by performing an arteriovenous fistula of the vein within the flap at the donor site for different periods of time before harvesting the arterialized venous flaps. Since then, pre-arterialization procedure as another promising technique was investigated to improve the survival of larger arterialized venous flaps by many authors. [21], [70], [71] Fukui et al [21] employed this technique by a two-week prearterialization to prevent congestion and necrosis of arterialized venous flaps using the model of rabbit ears with success. However, if a one-week pre-arterialization was performed, only slightly better results than in the standard arterialized venous flaps was achieved. Recently, Wungcharoe et al [72] noted that 7-day pre-arterialized flaps had no statistically significantly larger area of survival than arterialized venous flaps, and only the 14-day pre-arterialized flaps did. The mechanisms why pre-arterialized procedures improve the survival of arterialized venous flaps are still under investigation and its effects are inconsistent. A reasonable pre-arterialization period may play an important role on the improvement of the arterialized venous flaps. [30]

Recently, we performed an experimental study to investigate the improvement of the survival status of AVFs using pre-arterialization combined with delay procedure in rats. [73] We observed that the flaps in the group of pre-arterialization with delay procedure for one week achieved similar results as the conventional perfusion group. Vascular perfusion studies also revealed that the Indian ink filled the entire flaps in comparison with partially-filled flaps in other groups. This method may be a strategy for flap prefabrication based on the venous network.

8.3. Technique of noncontiguous and dual venous drainage

The reasons why the survival of AVFs is inconsistent are mainly attributed to the concerns of venous congestion. Rozen et al [74] introduced a modification in the design of saphenous venous flaps, whereby an arterialized flap is provided with a separate source of venous drainage that is not connected to the central vein-especially at the periphery of the flap for true venous drainage. There was a 0% complete flap loss rate (with only one case of superficial partial loss), and ultimately better survival than previous series of saphenous venous flaps described to date. The success of these techniques offers the potential to re-establish flow to large segmental losses to axial arteries, offer safe and definitive flap coverage to traumatic wounds, improve the array of flap options in this setting, and minimize donor site morbidity. [74] In Goldschlager et al's classification system [17], this technique was specifically emphasized.

Similarly, Lin et al [32] introduced a technique to improve flap survival following the similar concept using shunt-restricting approach. Shunt restriction was achieved in one of the following ways, according to the flap's venous pattern: (1) two parallel veins (II-pattern): use of separate veins for inflow and outflow; (2) two parallel veins with connecting branch (H-pattern): as for II-pattern, with ligation of connecting branch; (3) branching vein (Y/lambda-pattern): ligation of one branch near bifurcation, with use of that branch for outflow and other segment for inflow (or vice versa); and (4) one continuous vein (I-pattern): ligation at midpoint. A consecutive series of 15 flaps were transferred with the antegrade pattern. All flaps survived entirely with good outcomes comparable to conventional arterial flaps. Restriction of arterio-venous shunting enhances peripheral perfusion and decreases congestion of venous flaps, thereby improving reliability and utility in reconstructive surgery.

9. Summary

The arterialized venous flaps are easily designed and harvested with good quality. They are thin and pliable, without the need to sacrifice a major artery at the donor site, and no limitation of the donor site. They can be transferred not only as pure skin flaps, but also as composite flaps including tendons and nerves as well as vein grafts. Thus, the arterialized flaps are sometimes good candidates in reconstructive surgery, especially for the reconstruction of relatively small defects of hand and digits and have been useful tools in the plastic surgeons' armamentarium, which provide additional options in certain cases. Nonetheless, there is no consensus regarding their mechanism of survival or even the best approach to their design or transplantation, therefore, they do not completely replace the conventional flaps in plastic surgery and should be utilized in selected cases.

Author details

Hede Yan[1,2*], Cunyi Fan[2], Feng Zhang[3] and Weiyang Gao[1]

*Address all correspondence to: yanhede@hotmail.com

1 Department of Orthopedics (Division of Plastic and Hand Surgery), The Second Affiliated Hospital of Wenzhou Medical College, Wenzhou, China

2 Department of Orthopedics, The Sixth Affiliated People's Hospital, Shanghai Jiao Tong University, Shanghai, China

3 Division of Plastic Surgery, University of Mississippi Medical Center, Jackson, Mississippi, USA

References

[1] Nakayama, Y, Soeda, S, & Kasai, Y. Flaps nourished by arterial inflow through the venous system: an experimental investigation. *Plast Reconstr Surg.* Mar (1981). , 67(3), 328-334.

[2] Nishi, G, Shibata, Y, Kumabe, Y, Hattori, S, & Okuda, T. Arterialized venous skin flaps for the injured finger. *J Reconstr Microsurg.* Oct (1989). , 5(4), 357-365.

[3] Fasika, O. M, & Stilwell, J. H. Arterialized venous flap for covering and revascularizing finger injury. *Injury.* (1993). , 24(1), 67-68.

[4] Cheng, T. J, Chen, H. C, & Tang, Y. B. Salvage of a devascularized digit with free arterialized venous flap: a case report. *J Trauma.* Feb (1996). , 40(2), 308-310.

[5] Koch, H, Moshammer, H, Spendel, S, Pierer, G, & Scharnagl, E. Wrap-around arterialized venous flap for salvage of an avulsed finger. *J Reconstr Microsurg.* Jul (1999). , 15(5), 347-350.

[6] Inoue, G, & Tamura, Y. One-stage repair of both skin and tendon digital defects using the arterialized venous flap with palmaris longus tendon. *J Reconstr Microsurg.* Oct (1991). , 7(4), 339-343.

[7] Chen, C. L, Chiu, H. Y, Lee, J. W, & Yang, J. T. Arterialized tendocutaneous venous flap for dorsal finger reconstruction. *Microsurgery.* (1994). , 15(12), 886-890.

[8] Cho, B. C, Byun, J. S, & Baik, B. S. Dorsalis pedis tendocutaneous delayed arterialized venous flap in hand reconstruction. *Plast Reconstr Surg.* Dec (1999). , 104(7), 2138-2144.

[9] Kong, B. S, Kim, Y. J, Suh, Y. S, Jawa, A, Nazzal, A, & Lee, S. G. Finger soft tissue reconstruction using arterialized venous free flaps having 2 parallel veins. *J Hand Surg Am.* Dec (2008). , 33(10), 1802-1806.

[10] Yan, H, Zhang, F, & Akdemir, O. Clinical applications of venous flaps in the reconstruction of hands and fingers. *Arch Orthop Trauma Surg.* Jan (2011). , 131(1), 65-74.

[11] Yoshimura, M, Shimada, T, Imura, S, Shimamura, K, & Yamauchi, S. The venous skin graft method for repairing skin defects of the fingers. *Plast Reconstr Surg.* Feb (1987). , 79(2), 243-250.

[12] Tsai, T. M, Matiko, J. D, Breidenbach, W, & Kutz, J. E. Venous flaps in digital revascularization and replantation. *J Reconstr Microsurg.* Jan (1987). , 3(2), 113-119.

[13] Honda, T, Nomura, S, Yamauchi, S, Shimamura, K, & Yoshimura, M. The possible applications of a composite skin and subcutaneous vein graft in the replantation of amputated digits. *Br J Plast Surg.* Oct (1984). , 37(4), 607-612.

[14] Inoue, G, & Maeda, N. Arterialized venous flap coverage for skin defects of the hand or foot. *J Reconstr Microsurg.* Jul (1988)., 4(4), 259-266.

[15] De Lorenzi, F, & Van Der Hulst, R. R. den Dunnen WF, *et al.* Arterialized venous free flaps for soft-tissue reconstruction of digits: a 40-case series. *J Reconstr Microsurg.* Oct (2002). discussion 575-567., 18(7), 569-574.

[16] Nishi, G. Venous flaps for covering skin defects of the hand. *J Reconstr Microsurg.* Sep (1994)., 10(5), 313-319.

[17] Goldschlager, R, Rozen, W. M, Ting, J. W, & Leong, J. The nomenclature of venous flow-through flaps: Updated classification and review of the literature. *Microsurgery.* Sep (2012)., 32(6), 497-501.

[18] Lenoble, E, Foucher, G, Voisin, M. C, Maurel, A, & Goutallier, D. Observations on experimental flow-through venous flaps. *Br J Plast Surg.* Jul (1993)., 46(5), 378-383.

[19] Yuen, Q. M, & Leung, P. C. Some factors affecting the survival of venous flaps: an experimental study. *Microsurgery.* (1991)., 12(1), 60-64.

[20] Cho, B. C, Lee, M. S, Lee, J. H, Byun, J. S, & Baik, B. S. The effects of surgical and chemical delay procedures on the survival of arterialized venous flaps in rabbits. *Plast Reconstr Surg.* Sep (1998)., 102(4), 1134-1143.

[21] Fukui, A, Inada, Y, Murata, K, Ueda, Y, & Tamai, S. A method for prevention of arterialized venous flap necrosis. *J Reconstr Microsurg.* Jan (1998)., 14(1), 67-74.

[22] Byun, J. S, Constantinescu, M. A, Lee, W. P, & May, J. W. Jr. Effects of delay procedures on vasculature and survival of arterialized venous flaps: an experimental study in rabbits. *Plast Reconstr Surg.* Dec (1995)., 96(7), 1650-1659.

[23] Takato, T, Zuker, R. M, & Turley, C. B. Viability and versatility of arterialized venous perfusion flaps and prefabricated flaps: an experimental study in rabbits. *J Reconstr Microsurg.* Mar (1992)., 8(2), 111-119.

[24] Tan, M. P, Lim, A. Y, & Zhu, Q. A novel rabbit model for the evaluation of retrograde flow venous flaps. *Microsurgery.* (2009)., 29(3), 226-231.

[25] Xiu, Z. F, & Chen, Z. J. The microcirculation and survival of experimental flow-through venous flaps. *Br J Plast Surg.* Jan (1996)., 49(1), 41-45.

[26] Baek, S. M, Weinberg, H, Song, Y, Park, C. G, & Biller, H. F. Experimental studies in the survival of venous island flaps without arterial inflow. *Plast Reconstr Surg.* Jan (1985)., 75(1), 88-95.

[27] Germann, G. K, Eriksson, E, Russell, R. C, & Mody, N. Effect of arteriovenous flow reversal on blood flow and metabolism in a skin flap. *Plast Reconstr Surg.* Mar (1987)., 79(3), 375-380.

[28] Noreldin, A. A, Fukuta, K, & Jackson, I. T. Role of perivenous areolar tissue in the viability of venous flaps: an experimental study on the inferior epigastric venous flap of the rat. *Br J Plast Surg.* Jan (1992). , 45(1), 18-22.

[29] Shalaby, H. A, & Saad, M. A. The venous island flap: is it purely venous? *Br J Plast Surg.* Jun (1993). , 46(4), 285-287.

[30] Yan, H, Brooks, D, Ladner, R, Jackson, W. D, Gao, W, & Angel, M. F. Arterialized venous flaps: a review of the literature. *Microsurgery.* (2010). , 30(6), 472-478.

[31] Chen, H. C, Tang, Y. B, & Noordhoff, M. S. Four types of venous flaps for wound coverage: a clinical appraisal. *J Trauma.* Sep (1991). , 31(9), 1286-1293.

[32] Lin, Y. T, Henry, S. L, Lin, C. H, Lee, H. Y, Lin, W. N, & Wei, F. C. The shunt-restricted arterialized venous flap for hand/digit reconstruction: enhanced perfusion, decreased congestion, and improved reliability. *J Trauma.* Aug (2010). , 69(2), 399-404.

[33] Thatte, M. R, & Thatte, R. L. Venous flaps. *Plast Reconstr Surg.* Apr (1993). , 91(4), 747-751.

[34] Fukui, A, Inada, Y, Maeda, M, Mizumoto, S, Yajima, H, & Tamai, S. Venous flap--its classification and clinical applications. *Microsurgery.* (1994). , 15(8), 571-578.

[35] Woo, S. H, Kim, K. C, & Lee, G. J. A retrospective analysis of 154 arterialized venous flaps for hand reconstruction: an 11-year experience. *Plast Reconstr Surg.* May (2007). , 119(6), 1823-1838.

[36] Inoue, G, Maeda, N, & Suzuki, K. Resurfacing of skin defects of the hand using the arterialised venous flap. *Br J Plast Surg.* Mar (1990). , 43(2), 135-139.

[37] Brooks, D, Buntic, R, & Buncke, H. J. Use of a venous flap from an amputated part for salvage of an upper extremity injury. *Ann Plast Surg.* Feb (2002). , 48(2), 189-192.

[38] Yilmaz, M, Menderes, A, Karatas, O, Karaca, C, & Barutcu, A. Free arterialised venous forearm flaps for limb reconstruction. *Br J Plast Surg.* Sep (1996). , 49(6), 396-400.

[39] Woo, S. H, Jeong, J. H, & Seul, J. H. Resurfacing relatively large skin defects of the hand using arterialized venous flaps. *J Hand Surg Br.* Apr (1996). , 21(2), 222-229.

[40] Nakazawa, H, Nozaki, M, Kikuchi, Y, Honda, T, & Isago, T. Successful correction of severe contracture of the palm using arterialized venous flaps. *J Reconstr Microsurg.* Oct (2004). , 20(7), 527-531.

[41] Hyza, P, Vesely, J, Novak, P, Stupka, I, Sekac, J, & Choudry, U. Arterialized venous free flaps--a reconstructive alternative for large dorsal digital defects. *Acta Chir Plast.* (2008). , 50(2), 43-50.

[42] Inoue, G, & Suzuki, K. Arterialized venous flap for treating multiple skin defects of the hand. *Plast Reconstr Surg.* Feb (1993). discussion 303-296., 91(2), 299-302.

[43] Hyza, P, Vesely, J, Stupka, I, Cigna, E, & Monni, N. The bilobed arterialized venous free flap for simultaneous coverage of 2 separate defects of a digit. *Ann Plast Surg.* Dec (2005)., 55(6), 679-683.

[44] Trovato, M. J, Brooks, D, Buntic, R. F, & Buncke, G. M. Simultaneous coverage of two separate dorsal digital defects with a syndactylizing venous free flap. *Microsurgery.* (2008)., 28(4), 248-251.

[45] Nakazawa, H, Kikuchi, Y, Honda, T, Isago, T, Morioka, K, & Itoh, H. Use of an arterialised venous skin flap in the replantation of an amputated thumb. *Scand J Plast Reconstr Surg Hand Surg.* (2004)., 38(3), 187-191.

[46] Titley, O. G, & Chester, D. L. Park AJ. A-a type, arterialized, venous, flow-through, free flap for simultaneous digital revascularization and soft tissue reconstruction-revisited. *Ann Plast Surg.* Aug (2004)., 53(2), 185-191.

[47] Inoue, G, Tamura, Y, & Suzuki, K. One-stage repair of skin and tendon digital defects using the arterialized venous flap with palmaris longus tendon: an additional four cases. *J Reconstr Microsurg.* Feb (1996)., 12(2), 93-97.

[48] Yan, H F. C, Gao, W, Zhang, F, Li, Z, & Wang, C. Reconstruction of large dorsal digital defects with arterialized venous flaps: our experience and comprehensive review of literature. *Annals of Plastic Surgery.* (2012).

[49] Kayikcioglu, A, Akyurek, M, Safak, T, Ozkan, O, & Kecik, A. Arterialized venous dorsal digital island flap for fingertip reconstruction. *Plast Reconstr Surg.* Dec (1998). discussion 2373., 102(7), 2368-2372.

[50] Takeuchi, M, Sakurai, H, Sasaki, K, & Nozaki, M. Treatment of finger avulsion injuries with innervated arterialized venous flaps. *Plast Reconstr Surg.* Sep (2000)., 106(4), 881-885.

[51] Yan, H, Gao, W, Zhang, F, Li, Z, Chen, X, & Fan, C. A comparative study of finger pulp reconstruction using arterialised venous sensate flap and insensate flap from forearm. *J Plast Reconstr Aesthet Surg.* Sep (2012)., 65(9), 1220-1226.

[52] Kushima, H, Iwasawa, M, & Maruyama, Y. Recovery of sensitivity in the hand after reconstruction with arterialised venous flaps. *Scand J Plast Reconstr Surg Hand Surg.* (2002)., 36(6), 362-367.

[53] Chia, J, Lim, A, & Peng, Y. P. Use of an arterialized venous flap for resurfacing a circumferential soft tissue defect of a digit. *Microsurgery.* (2001)., 21(8), 374-378.

[54] Brooks, D, Buntic, R. F, & Taylor, C. Use of the venous flap for salvage of difficult ring avulsion injuries. *Microsurgery.* (2008)., 28(6), 397-402.

[55] Iwasawa, M, Ohtsuka, Y, Kushima, H, & Kiyono, M. Arterialized venous flaps from the thenar and hypothenar regions for repairing finger pulp tissue losses. *Plast Reconstr Surg.* May (1997)., 99(6), 1765-1770.

[56] Yokoyama, T, Cardaci, A, Hosaka, Y, Revol, M, Alcontres, d, & Servant, F. S. JM. Location of communicating veins for medial plantar venous flap. *Ann Plast Surg.* Jul (2008)., 61(1), 99-104.

[57] Yokoyama, T, Hosaka, Y, Servant, J. M, Takagi, S, & Cardaci, A. A simplification for harvesting medial plantar venous flap with communicating veins: usefulness of preoperative ultrasound imaging. *Ann Plast Surg.* Apr (2008)., 60(4), 379-385.

[58] Yokoyama, T, Tosa, Y, Hashikawa, M, Kadota, S, & Hosaka, Y. Medial plantar venous flap technique for volar oblique amputation with no defects in the nail matrix and nail bed. *J Plast Reconstr Aesthet Surg.* Nov (2010)., 63(11), 1870-1874.

[59] (Lille S, Brown RE, Zook EE, Russell RC. Free nonvascularized composite nail grafts: an institutional experience. Plast Reconstr Surg. Jun 2000;105(7):2412-2415). 105(7), 2412-2415.

[60] Nakayama, Y, Iino, T, Uchida, A, Kiyosawa, T, & Soeda, S. Vascularized free nail grafts nourished by arterial inflow from the venous system. *Plast Reconstr Surg.* Feb (1990). discussion 246-237., 85(2), 239-245.

[61] Kovacs, A. F. Comparison of two types of arterialized venous forearm flaps for oral reconstruction and proposal of a reliable procedure. *J Craniomaxillofac Surg.* Aug (1998)., 26(4), 249-254.

[62] Iglesias, M, Butron, P, Chavez-munoz, C, Ramos-sanchez, I, & Barajas-olivas, A. Arterialized venous free flap for reconstruction of burned face. *Microsurgery.* (2008)., 28(7), 546-550.

[63] Park, S. W, Heo, E. P, & Choi, J. H. Reconstruction of defects after excision of facial skin cancer using a venous free flap. *Ann Plast Surg.* Dec (2011)., 67(6), 608-611.

[64] Inada, Y, Hirai, T, Fukui, A, Omokawa, S, Mii, Y, & Tamai, S. An experimental study of the flow-through venous flap: investigation of the width and area of survival with one flow-through vein preserved. *J Reconstr Microsurg.* Jul (1992)., 8(4), 297-302.

[65] Kakinoki, R, Ikeguchi, R, Nankaku, M, & Nakamua, T. Factors affecting the success of arterialised venous flaps in the hand. *Injury.* Oct (2008). Suppl, 4, 18-24.

[66] Moshammer, H. E, Schwarzl, F. X, & Haas, F. M. Retrograde arterialized venous flap: an experimental study. *Microsurgery.* (2003)., 23(2), 130-134.

[67] Koch, H, Scharnagl, E, Schwarzl, F. X, Haas, F. M, Hubmer, M, & Moshammer, H. E. Clinical application of the retrograde arterialized venous flap. *Microsurgery.* (2004)., 24(2), 118-124.

[68] Morris, S. F, & Taylor, G. I. The time sequence of the delay phenomenon: when is a surgical delay effective? An experimental study. *Plast Reconstr Surg.* Mar (1995)., 95(3), 526-533.

[69] Cho, B. C, Lee, J. H, Byun, J. S, & Baik, B. S. Clinical applications of the delayed arterialized venous flap. *Ann Plast Surg.* Aug (1997)., 39(2), 145-157.

[70] Alexander, G. Multistage type III venous flap or'pre-arterialisation of an arterialised venous flap'. *Br J Plast Surg.* Dec (2001).

[71] Wungcharoen, B, Santidhananon, Y, & Chongchet, V. Pre-arterialisation of an arterialised venous flap: clinical cases. *Br J Plast Surg.* Mar (2001)., 54(2), 112-116.

[72] Wungcharoen, B, Pradidarcheep, W, Santidhananon, Y, & Chongchet, V. Pre-arterialisation of the arterialised venous flap: an experimental study in the rat. *Br J Plast Surg.* Oct (2001)., 54(7), 621-630.

[73] Yan, H, Brooks, D, Jackson, W. D, Angel, M. F, Akdemir, O, & Zhang, F. Improvement of prearterialized venous flap survival with delay procedure in rats. *J Reconstr Microsurg.* Apr (2010)., 26(3), 193-200.

[74] Rozen, W. M, Ting, J. W, Gilmour, R. F, & Leong, J. The arterialized saphenous venous flow-through flap with dual venous drainage. *Microsurgery.* May (2012)., 32(4), 281-288.